T0146291

Managed Care

and the

Evaluation and
Adoption of

Emerging
Medical
Technologies

Steven Garber ◆ M. Susan Ridgely ◆ Roger S. Taylor ◆ Robin Meili

Supported by the Health Industry Manufacturers Association,
the California Goldstrike Partnership, and the U.S. Economic Development Administration

RAND

The research described in this report was supported by the Health Industry Manufacturers Association, the Goldstrike Partnership—a program of the California Trade and Commerce Agency's Office of Strategic Technology—and the Economic Development Administration of the U.S. Department of Commerce.

ISBN: 0-8330-2831-6

This publication was prepared by RAND for the California Trade and Commerce Agency's Office of Strategic Technology and the Health Industry Manufacturers Association. The statements, conclusions, and recommendations are those of the author(s) and do not necessarily reflect the views of the Economic Development Administration.

Published 2000 by RAND
1700 Main Street, P.O. Box 2138, Santa Monica, CA 90407-2138
1333 H St., N.W., Washington, D.C. 20005-4707
RAND URL: http://www.rand.org/
To order RAND documents or to obtain additional information,
contact Distribution Services: Telephone: (310) 451-7002;
Fax: (310) 451-6915; Internet: order@rand.org

New medical technologies—pharmaceuticals, medical devices, and procedures—often allow great improvements in the outcomes of medical care, but they are also widely believed to be a major cause of increasing costs. *Selective adoption of new technologies,* the taking on of only those technologies for which the medical benefits exceed the costs to society of developing and using them, is a crucial element in the quest to control health care costs while preserving or enhancing the quality of care.

This report focuses on adoption of innovative medical technologies by managed care organizations (MCOs). The project had two primary objectives: (1) to understand current processes MCOs use for making coverage, medical-necessity, and payment decisions involving emerging medical technologies, and how device developers and manufacturers prepare for and participate in these processes; and (2) to identify ways that private, voluntary action by the managed-care and medical-device industries individually or jointly might improve—for the benefit of society—the processes by which new medical technologies are developed, evaluated, and adopted or rejected for coverage.

We gathered empirical information from in-depth, semi-structured interviews with eight manufacturers of innovative devices and nine managed care organizations. We also collected information from representatives of manufacturers, MCOs, and the sponsors of this study—the California Goldstrike Partnership, the Economic Development Administration of the U.S. Department of Commerce, and the Health Industry Manufacturers Association (HIMA)—at a half-day, invitation-only meeting held at RAND headquarters on October 7, 1999.

The most novel aspect of the study is collection of extensive information from manufacturers and juxtaposition of their reported experiences and perspectives with those of MCOs. We had four primary audiences in mind when conducting this research and reporting our findings: medical-device developers and manufacturers, managed care organizations, public-policy makers, and researchers and analysts. Members of all four audiences will find something of interest here. Experienced device manufacturers—i.e., companies that have already marketed devices in the United States—may, for example, be spurred to think about marketing to MCOs in new ways. Aspiring device manufacturers—i.e., organizations that are attempting to develop innovative devices but that have no experience in marketing such products—and their investors may learn the most. In particular, many observers believe that such organizations often fail to look past Food and Drug Administration approval of their products to the challenges they will face in the marketplace, and find themselves inadequately prepared for the commercialization effort. Likewise, as MCOs attempt to make numerous difficult decisions regarding emerging technologies, they are likely to benefit from considering the perspectives of manufacturers and the processes and perspectives of other MCOs. Public policies can influence MCO technology-adoption decisions for privately insured consumers. It would be beneficial, then, for policymakers to consider how their decisions may affect medical innovation indirectly through the effects of those decisions on private technology adoption, along with the more obvious direct effects of their decisions about coverage and payment under public health insurance programs. In addition, government agencies concerned with job creation and economic development should be interested in our findings concerning determinants of commercial success for medical-technology developers and manufacturers. Finally, researchers and analysts may be interested in various issues discussed here, such as decisionmaking by MCOs, device manufacturers' commercialization strategies and tactics, how the interaction of the two determines demand for emerging medical technologies, and the nature of incentives for medical innovation.

This report is based on research conducted under the auspices of RAND Health. RAND Health furthers RAND's mission of helping improve policy and decisionmaking through research and analysis, by working to improve health care systems and advance understanding of how the organization and financing of care affect costs, quality, and access.

CONTENTS

Appendix

New medical technologies—pharmaceuticals, medical devices, and procedures—often allow major improvements in the outcomes of medical care, but they are also widely believed to be a leading cause of increasing costs. Selective adoption of new technologies, the taking on of only those technologies for which the medical benefits exceed the costs to society of developing and using them, is a crucial element in the quest to control health care costs while preserving or enhancing the quality of care.

This report focuses on adoption of innovative medical technologies by managed care organizations (MCOs). The project had two primary objectives: (1) to understand current processes of MCOs for making coverage, medical-necessity, and payment decisions involving emerging medical technologies, and how device developers and manufacturers prepare for and participate in these processes; and (2) to identify ways that private, voluntary action by the managed-care and device industries individually or jointly might improve—for the benefit of society—the processes by which new medical technologies are developed, evaluated, and adopted or rejected for coverage.

Extensive information about MCO processes was collected through confidential, in-depth interviews with eight manufacturers of innovative medical devices and medical directors of nine California MCOs, five of which are affiliated with national MCOs. The preliminary findings from these interviews were presented at a meeting on October 7, 1999, at which representatives of manufacturers, MCOs, and the sponsoring organizations—the State of California's Goldstrike Partnership, the Economic Development Administration of the U.S. Department of Commerce, and the Health Industry Manufacturers Association—critiqued and elaborated on our findings and interpretations. The study is especially novel in collecting and synthesizing information about the experiences and perspectives of manufacturers, and in juxtaposing their reported experiences and perspectives with those of MCOs.

PERSPECTIVES OF MANUFACTURERS

We sought to interview individuals at companies that are actively marketing medical devices that might offer significant medical advances over alternatives but that also might increase costs to MCOs. Each interview addressed four sets of issues:

- Background on the company and the one or two devices on which the interview focused

- The experience of the company in marketing the device or devices to MCOs

- Factors other than MCO behavior affecting adoption of the technology

- Lessons learned and advice for somewhat inexperienced device developers and manufacturers.

Part of the second goal of the project was to develop information that could help manufacturers understand the market environment and to prepare accordingly. Almost all of the interview subjects emphasized early development of commercialization strategies and planning for commercialization efforts. Virtually all manufacturers emphasized that, well before a product is ready for Food and Drug Administration (FDA) review, companies should analyze various issues, including the following:

- Prevalence, incidence, and patient demographics of the disease or medical condition at which the product is aimed

- Effectiveness, safety, and costs of existing alternatives to the product

- Availability and levels of reimbursement for similar devices

- Reimbursement codes and reimbursement levels for professional and institutional services associated with the product

- Importance of Medicare coverage for the prospective patients.

Almost all interview subjects emphasized early planning of clinical and economic studies. In this regard, subjects suggested that the following steps be taken:

- When planning studies, ask payers what kind of information they would find useful in making coverage and medical-necessity decisions.

- Develop clear, evidence-based guidelines for appropriate use.

- Develop evidence that the FDA does not require for product approval.

- Work with centers of excellence in designing and executing studies.

- Involve in the studies influential physicians who may become champions of the technologies.

- Make sure, however, that those studies that are undertaken are good investments.

PERSPECTIVES OF MCO MEDICAL DIRECTORS

To understand how MCOs respond to the availability of new medical technologies, we sought to interview managed care organizations representing a substantial proportion of the managed care market in California. Each interview addressed five sets of issues:

- The extent of formal technology assessments of new medical devices, the processes employed, and the role of manufacturers

- How the MCO makes coverage decisions for procedures involving emerging medical devices

- How the MCO sets payment or reimbursement levels for medical devices

- How case-by-case medical-necessity determinations are made

- Lessons learned and advice for medical device manufacturers.

All of the interview subjects emphasized that technology adoption for MCOs involves a multilayered process for determining whether a procedure, and any devices involved, will be eligible for payment. Within that process of coverage decisionmaking, formal technology-assessment processes vary widely across MCOs with respect to

- The level of formality, including whether the MCO uses staff in addition to the medical director and one or more standing committees to conduct the technology assessment

- Who is responsible for decisionmaking

- The rigor—depth and breadth—of the review of medical evidence

- The use of outside expertise and resources, including technology-assessment firms and national or local physician experts

- The extent to which MCOs are influenced by governmental organizations and health-insurance-industry leaders

- The average number of formal technology reviews conducted each year.

Technology assessment is usually a closed process, and manufacturers are not allowed to participate directly. Yet MCOs report that they consider information supplied by manufacturers and, while carefully reviewing the design and methodology, accord the same weight to manufacturer-sponsored, peer-reviewed studies as they do to other peer-reviewed studies.

There were varying levels of enthusiasm for joint efforts between manufacturers and MCOs. At least one MCO medical director offered each of the following suggestions:

- Manufacturers should help MCOs anticipate what technologies are "in the pipeline" and the potential costs.

- Manufacturers should share information on experience with medical devices across MCOs and providers.

- Manufacturers and MCOs should foster cooperative research in routine clinical settings.

- Manufacturers and MCOs should facilitate cooperative provider education.

- Manufacturers and MCOs should create contracts that enable the MCOs to upgrade expensive, multi-use devices as improvements are made.

- MCOs should allow manufacturers to participate in technology assessment processes.

HOW MIGHT TECHNOLOGY ADOPTION BE IMPROVED?

The social goal of adopting or rejecting technologies on the basis of their social costs and benefits involves enormous complexities and uncertainties, and achieving anything close to perfection in winnowing technologies is not possible. However, in view of the size of the U.S. health care system and of the potential contributions of new technology to health, even incremental improvements could have large payoffs.

A major impediment to socially appropriate adoption of emerging medical technologies is limited information about the performance of these technologies—both absolutely and relative to alternative technologies—in day-to-day medical practice. We see prospects for improving four elements of information availability:

- Developing better information before market introduction

- Learning more from experience after market introduction

- Evaluating and synthesizing clinical information

- Disseminating information.

We also discuss several other issues that warrant consideration:

- Aligning private incentives of MCOs and payers with social values

- Enhancing MCO capabilities to evaluate technologies and make decisions

- Improving decisions by physicians
- Reducing use of inappropriate or obsolete technologies
- Reducing costs of decisionmaking for manufacturers and MCOs
- Improving manufacturer understanding of the market environment
- Helping MCOs and employers anticipate what is in the pipeline.

Improving the processes of medical-technology adoption raises numerous, complex issues. The discussion at the October 7 meeting provided reason to hope that representatives of the managed-care and medical-technology industries could engage in constructive, joint exploration of what might be accomplished by private, voluntary action. It was also agreed that it would be very helpful to include payers (e.g., consortia of employers) in such a process. Various issues raised above provide potential agenda items for such discussions.

The research reported here was sponsored by the Health Industry Manufacturers Association (HIMA) with funds provided by the Goldstrike Partnership—a program of the California Trade and Commerce Agency's Office of Strategic Technology—and the Economic Development Administration (EDA) of the U.S. Department of Commerce. We are indebted to several individuals associated with these organizations for aiding our efforts in various ways. Specifically, we thank Pam Bailey (HIMA), Alex Glass (Bay Area Regional Technology Alliance), Maxene Johnston (Johnston and Company), Candace Littell (C.L. & Associates), Jeff Newman (Office of Strategic Technology, California Trade and Commerce Agency), Dee Simons (HIMA), Leonard Smith (EDA), and Deena Sosson (EDA).

We are also indebted to dozens of people who generously provided information that represents the core data used in our analysis. They include individuals at eight companies that manufacture medical devices and nine managed care organizations (MCOs) who participated in confidential interviews and several representatives of manufacturers and MCOs who participated in a meeting held at RAND on October 7, 1999, during which our preliminary findings were critiqued and discussed and additional information was collected. Owing to our pledges of confidentiality, we cannot thank these individuals by name.

We also thank Meg Bernhardt and Dotty Marsh of RAND for helping to arrange interviews and the October 7 meeting. RAND colleagues Rebecca D'Amato and Elizabeth Rolph generously shared notes on literature concerning coverage decisionmaking by health plans.

Finally, we thank our technical reviewers—Katherine Harris of RAND and Scott D. Ramsey of the University of Washington—for timely, thoughtful, and constructive comments and suggestions.

Chapter One

INTRODUCTION

PROJECT BACKGROUND AND OBJECTIVES

Health policy analysts and policymakers often struggle with conflicting views about the development and adoption of new pharmaceuticals, medical devices, and procedures. Society looks to technological advances to improve the quality and outcomes of medical care. Although new technologies sometimes enable improved quality with lower costs, new technology is often viewed as a major cause of increasing costs of health care in the United States.[1]

Knowledgeable, reasonable participants and observers disagree about the extent to which new medical technology affects health and health care costs. But most agree in principle that the well-being of society as a whole is improved when health-care providers adopt those new technologies whose contributions to health warrant any additional costs and reject technologies—old and new—that do not satisfy this criterion. A collection of processes that effectively winnows technologies in this fashion would also send a socially valuable message to aspiring inventors and innovators: Technologies that serve the social good are likely to be rewarded in the marketplace; other technologies are not. Making socially desirable technology-adoption decisions and sending clear signals to inventors, innovators, and investors are, of course, much easier said than done. However, the enormous health and economic stakes suggest that even minor improvements over current practices of technology de-

---

[1]See, for example, Weisbrod (1991) and Newhouse (1993).

velopment, marketing, and adoption could be well worth the costs of achieving them.

The project on which we report here had two primary objectives: (1) to understand current processes of managed care organizations (MCOs) for making coverage, medical-necessity, and payment decisions involving emerging medical technologies, and how device developers and manufacturers prepare for and participate in these processes; and (2) to identify ways that private, voluntary action by the managed-care and device industries, individually or jointly, might improve—for the benefit of society—the processes by which new medical technologies are developed, evaluated, and adopted or rejected for coverage. We focus on decisions and actions by medical device manufacturers and managed care organizations regarding coverage of and payment for innovative medical devices and related medical procedures. We refer to such devices and procedures as "emerging medical technologies" to connote that these technologies have as yet been neither widely adopted nor widely rejected in the marketplace. We define *managed care organizations* broadly to include both health plans (such as health maintenance organizations) and medical groups that contract with health plans to provide care to patients on a capitated basis or through other arrangements that place the groups at financial risk.

Managed care uses various organizational forms and management techniques to try to control costs while preserving or enhancing the quality of care. These efforts affect the processes and outcomes of technology adoption. Management of care per se is not problematic; the earlier approach of generally paying for whatever physicians and patients requested when someone else was bearing the costs left much to be desired. The critical questions are how well managed care currently handles technology adoption and how improvements that benefit society at large might be achieved.[2] In light of the ongo-

---

[2]Goddeeris (1984a,b), Baumgardner (1991), and Ramsey and Pauly (1997) present formal theoretical analyses of how health insurance arrangements can affect technology adoption. Goddeeris (1984a,b) and Baumgardner (1991) conclude that insurance can lead to technology adoption that makes society as a whole worse off. Baumgardner shows how different approaches to cost control (i.e., traditional fee-for-service with coinsurance, and a prepaid health plan without coinsurance but with institutional restrictions on treatment levels) are vulnerable to inefficiencies from different types of technological change. Ramsey and Pauly (1997) incorporate the ability of

ing and intense public debate over managed care, proposals for expanded federal and state regulation, and the widespread public interest in medical innovation, investigating how managed care affects medical-technology adoption is particularly timely.

OVERVIEW OF THE STUDY

Our work contributes to—and begins to fill some significant gaps in—a growing literature on technology adoption in the U.S. health care marketplace. Previous studies include econometric analyses of adoption of specific medical technologies[3] and of decisionmaking by health plans based on interviews or mail surveys designed to probe determinants of adoption of specific medical technologies or medical technology broadly construed. Our study focuses on innovative medical devices and related procedures. We gathered empirical information from in-depth, semi-structured interviews with eight manufacturers of innovative devices and nine managed care organizations. We also collected information from representatives of manufacturers, MCOs, and the sponsors of this study—the California Goldstrike Partnership,[4] the Economic Development Administration of the U.S. Department of Commerce, and the Health Industry Manufacturers Association (HIMA)[5]—at a half-day, invitation-only meeting held at RAND headquarters on October 7, 1999.[6] At this meeting, we presented the preliminary findings from our interviews, and participants were encouraged to critique and elaborate. The study is especially novel in collecting extensive information from manufacturers and in juxtaposing their reported experiences and perspectives with those of MCOs.

---

fee-for-service plans to control use of new technologies and conclude that Health Maintenance Organizations (HMOs) may adopt some costly technologies that are not adopted under fee-for-service arrangements and vice versa.

[3]Baker and Wheeler (1998) and Spetz and Baker (1999) and studies cited in them.

[4]The Goldstrike Partnership is a program of the California Trade and Commerce Agency's Office of Strategic Technology.

[5]HIMA is a trade association based in Washington, D.C. It represents more than 800 manufacturers of medical devices, diagnostic products, and medical information systems.

[6]Some of the manufacturers and MCOs that participated in interviews also sent representatives to the meeting, and others did not. Many of the manufacturers and MCOs represented at the meeting had not participated as interview subjects.

In conducting this research and reporting our findings, we had four primary audiences in mind:

- Medical device developers and manufacturers

- Managed care organizations

- Public-policy makers

- Researchers and analysts.

Members of all four audiences are likely to find something of interest here. Experienced device manufacturers—i.e., companies that have already marketed devices in the United States—may, for example, be spurred to think about marketing to MCOs in new ways. Aspiring device manufacturers—i.e., organizations that are attempting to develop innovative devices but have no experience in marketing such products—and their investors may learn the most. In particular, many observers believe that such organizations often fail to look past Food and Drug Administration (FDA) approval of their products to the challenges they will face in the marketplace, and then find themselves poorly prepared for the commercialization effort. As a consequence, they may perform less well for themselves and their employees, investors, communities, and potential consumers than if they had been more forward-looking.[7]

Likewise, as MCOs attempt to make numerous difficult decisions regarding emerging technologies, they are likely to benefit from considering the perspectives of manufacturers and the processes and perspectives of other MCOs. Public policies[8] can influence MCO technology-adoption decisions for privately insured consumers. It would be beneficial, then, for policymakers to consider how their

---

[7]In fact, concerns of this sort motivated the Goldstrike Partnership and the Economic Development Administration to provide financial support for this project. More specifically: "The changing dynamics in the healthcare delivery system and increasing penetration of managed care organizations has changed the way business is done in this arena. Most new technology companies are unprepared to address the new dynamics in this industry and need assistance in dealing with these critical commercialization issues" (Johnston and Company, 1998).

[8]Such as coverage and reimbursement policies of the Health Care Financing Administration (HCFA) and technology assessments supported and disseminated by the Agency for Healthcare Research and Quality (AHRQ) (formerly the Agency for Health Care Policy and Research, or AHCPR).

decisions may affect medical innovation indirectly through their effects on technology adoption and incentives to innovate, along with the more obvious direct effects of their decisions about coverage and payment under public health insurance programs. In addition, government agencies concerned with job creation and economic development should be interested in our findings concerning determinants of commercial success for medical-technology developers and manufacturers. Finally, researchers and analysts may be interested in various issues discussed below, such as decisionmaking by MCOs, device manufacturers' commercialization strategies and tactics, how the interaction of the two determines demand for emerging medical technologies, and the nature of incentives for medical innovation.

The remainder of this report comprises five chapters. For the convenience of our diverse audiences, the main text is written to be accessible to nonresearchers; details and technical material—including guides to related literature—are presented in footnotes. In Chapter Two, we briefly describe steps that can be involved in determining MCO coverage for a particular technology. In Chapters Three and Four, we summarize and interpret what we were told in our interviews with manufacturers and managed care organizations, respectively. In Chapter Five, we present advice offered by the two sets of interview respondents for consideration by device manufacturers as they decide how to invest in medical technology development and plan commercialization efforts. In the concluding chapter, Chapter Six, we step back to consider implications of the interviews, the discussion at the October 7 meeting, and the literature and discuss key challenges for improving the processes of evaluating and adopting or rejecting medical devices and the medical procedures employing them.

Much of the value of the information we present requires recognition of the variety of clinical and economic contexts of emerging medical technologies and the wide range of factors that determine the outcomes of commercialization efforts. We hope that the information offered here enables readers to develop an enhanced understanding of our highly complex and varied technology-adoption system. If so, it may aid readers as they pursue their distinct objectives, and contribute to the social goals of balancing health care costs and quality and providing socially appropriate signals to guide investments in medical innovation.

Chapter Two

TECHNOLOGY-ADOPTION DECISIONS BY MCOs: AN OVERVIEW

This chapter provides a general background, culled from the literature and our interviews, for the discussions that follow. It describes basic issues and activities that can be involved in technology-adoption decisions by MCOs. As will become apparent, decision processes are often much less orderly than might be inferred from this general overview, and the processes that are used vary both across MCOs and within MCOs, depending on the particular technology or context.

For a technology to be eligible for payment or reimbursement by a managed care organization, usually the technology must not be excluded by the language of the health insurance contract between the MCO and payers,[1] which generally means that the technology must contribute to provision of one of the broad categories of services specified as being covered (e.g., hospital services, physician office visits, durable medical equipment), must be "medically necessary" under the particular circumstances of the case,[2] and must not be "experimental" or "investigational."[3] In addition, many contracts

---

[1]Sometimes care is provided despite contractual limitations, e.g., for fear of legal action. See, for example, Hall and Anderson (1992), Anderson (1992), Anderson et al. (1993), Ferguson et al. (1993), Havighurst (1995), and Adler (1996).

[2]See, for example, Havighurst (1995, pp. 125–132).

[3]See, for example, Havighurst (1995, pp. 132–135). Medical devices are generally considered experimental or investigational prior to FDA approval for U.S. marketing, and may be considered experimental or investigational for all or selected uses well after approval.

exclude or limit coverage for various more or less specific services.[4] The contractual framework is typically determined through negotiations between purchasers (e.g., employers) and personnel operating on the business or marketing side of an MCO.

Within this framework, MCO personnel, such as a medical director and utilization review staff, interpret contracts to make decisions about coverage and payment for emerging technologies. Sometimes an MCO undertakes a formal process to determine whether a technology should be covered under any circumstance. Such decisions can require judgments about whether the technology pertains to a covered benefit or is investigational, or about the conditions under which its use is safe and effective. Many of these issues can be informed by a "technology assessment." Precisely what different people mean by this term varies. Generally, the term is used to describe somewhat structured efforts to judge the clinical effectiveness, and sometimes also the cost-effectiveness, of medical technologies. *Technology assessment* usually involves critical evaluation and synthesis of evidence available from clinical studies and other systematic evidence; often, expert opinion is incorporated.[5]

If medical directors, committees, or other staff determine that a technology is covered, patient-selection criteria are often developed. Broadly speaking, these criteria specify the circumstances under which use of the technology is viewed as medically necessary. These criteria guide decisions about eligibility of particular patients for coverage—for example, in response to requests for pre-authorization (i.e., a commitment by the MCO to pay) from a physician who wants to use the technology.

---

[4]For example, contracts often exclude "dental care, sexual reassignment surgery, in vitro fertilization, reversal of voluntary sterilization, treatment for morbid obesity, and cosmetic surgery solely for the purposes of beautification . . ."(Havighurst, 1995, p. 141, fn. 19). See Booske (1994) for a very detailed analysis of provisions for covered benefits, coverage exclusions, limitations on use, and cost-sharing specified in contracts between health insurers and state employees in several states.

[5]*Technology assessment* has been defined by one author as "the evaluation of the safety, effectiveness, and appropriateness of the many devices, medical and surgical procedures, and pharmaceuticals promoted to improve a patient's condition or quality of life" (Matuszewski, 1997). This report focuses more narrowly on technology assessment of medical devices and related procedures. Rettig (1997) studies technology assessment for pharmaceuticals, procedures, and devices. For studies of technology assessment of pharmaceuticals, see Lyles et al. (1997).

Chapter Three

HOW DEVICE MANUFACTURERS SEE THE SYSTEM

In this chapter, we describe and interpret what we were told in interviews with representatives of eight companies that manufacture and market innovative medical devices. We begin by providing background on how companies were selected and recruited to participate, the issues addressed in the interviews, and the companies and devices on which the interviews focused. We then report and interpret what we were told about the recent experiences of the companies in marketing their devices to managed care organizations. In accordance with our pledge of confidentiality to interview respondents, the discussion is somewhat general in order to avoid inadvertently revealing the identity of any participating manufacturer. Nevertheless, we believe we convey an informative depiction of many aspects of the market environment as perceived by the interview respondents.

BACKGROUND ON MANUFACTURER INTERVIEWS

Recruitment of Interview Respondents

A critical issue confronting health care delivery in the United States is the tension between controlling cost and promoting quality of care. To enable us to learn about how this tension may play out in the context of emerging medical technologies, we sought to interview companies actively marketing medical devices

- whose commercial fate could depend on decisions of MCOs[1]

- that differ from predecessor devices in ways that might offer significant medical advantages

- whose use might involve higher MCO costs than those of alternative approaches to the same therapeutic or diagnostic goal.

Given the interests of the sponsoring California Goldstrike Partnership, we also made a special effort to include companies based in, or with substantial operations in, California. Candidate devices and the companies were identified in various ways, including review of FDA lists of recently approved devices, review of trade press, and discussions with staff of HIMA.

Once companies of interest were identified, HIMA staff made initial contact with those companies that are HIMA members. If these contacts elicited sufficient interest, a RAND investigator followed up to explain the project and request an interview. Five interviews were arranged through this route. For those non–HIMA-member companies identified as appropriate to the project goals, recruitment was handled entirely by RAND project staff. This approach added two interviews. Finally, three companies contacted HIMA upon hearing about the study, to volunteer for interviews. One of them met our criteria and was included in the sample. In all cases, when RAND contacted a company to request an interview, we faxed a description of the project and its goals (Appendix A) and a description of the interview, including a list of interview questions (Appendix B). When requesting an interview, we suggested a particular device for discussion—specifically, the device that led us to request an interview—and invited companies to suggest a second.

Content of Interviews

As detailed in Appendix B, the interviews with manufacturers addressed four sets of issues:

---

[1]Which excludes, for example, various types of equipment that are marketed directly to and purchased by hospitals.

- Background on the company and the one or two devices on which the interview focused

- The experience of the company in marketing the device or devices to MCOs

- Factors other than MCO behavior affecting adoption of the technology

- Lessons learned and advice for largely inexperienced device developers and manufacturers.

All of the companies that agreed to interviews also agreed to discuss the device that led us to approach them. In two cases, a second device that was suggested by the interview respondent was discussed as well. The number of interview respondents per company varied from one (in four cases) to three. In two cases, the only, or lead, respondent was a corporate vice president. Otherwise, he or she was a director or manager of reimbursement or product manager for the device on which the interview focused. Two of the interviews were conducted in person; six were conducted by telephone.

The planned duration of the interviews was 60 to 90 minutes, but almost all of them lasted 90 minutes or more. Interview respondents were promised confidentiality, were told they were free to tell us that a subject was too sensitive to be discussed, and were encouraged to point out information that was particularly sensitive. While respondents often provided information that was proprietary and, on occasion, identified information as especially sensitive, they seemed to be very candid and forthcoming. Questions were rarely deflected because they were too sensitive to discuss.

Descriptions of Companies Interviewed and Devices Discussed

Most of the companies are publicly held. They range in size from very small to large (e.g., a few dozen to several thousand employees). Almost all of them focus on developing, manufacturing, and marketing medical devices. The proportion of the companies' R&D and manufacturing activity located in California runs the gamut from none to virtually all. Three of the companies are based in California.

For half of the companies, a device on which the interview focused was the company's only or key commercial product. All but one of the devices discussed is for therapeutic use.[2] The indications for use varied widely, including life-threatening acute or chronic conditions, traumatic injury, or physical disability. Three of the devices are permanently implanted, two are used for drug delivery, and two promote healing of wounds. The populations of potential users in the United States annually ranged from roughly ten thousand to several million. The devices were approved for use by the U.S. Food and Drug Administration as early as the 1980s and as recently as 1997.[3] One device discussed at length, in parallel with another product of the same company, had not yet been approved by the FDA.[4]

All of the devices discussed met our criterion of involving significant potential costs per patient. In some cases, the price of the device represents a majority of the cost of using the technology; in others, the cost of the associated procedure accounts for a majority of the costs. The prices of the devices ranged from a few thousand to many thousands of dollars per patient. The per-patient costs of related professional services, such as surgery, hospitalization, and post-

---

[2]One of the interviews focused on a somewhat unusual diagnostic device; to discuss it further could enable some readers to identify the product.

[3]Most new medical devices require FDA approval to be marketed in the United States. There is no analogous regulatory process for reviewing medical procedures. To gain access to the market, high-risk (Class III) medical devices are subject to an FDA review process—specifically, of a pre-market approval application (PMA)—that requires submission of results of clinical trials demonstrating safety and efficacy. Much larger numbers of devices that are thought to be less risky reach the market through the less-demanding 510(k) pre-market notification process, which requires a device to be "substantially equivalent" to a legally marketed device. The FDA sometimes requires submission of clinical evidence before approving 510(k) applications, which blurs the distinction between the two processes. In fact, Merrill (1994), who provides a detailed description of FDA regulation of medical devices, argues that the FDA has been steadily moving toward the "drug model" of regulation for devices, thereby thwarting the intent of Congress to foster device innovation. For more-detailed descriptions of FDA regulation of medical devices, see Gibbs and Mackler (1987), Garber (1993, pp. 29–31), Wholey and Haller (1995), National Health Policy Forum (1998, pp. 4–5), and Ramsey et al. (1998).

[4]The interviews did not emphasize issues pertaining to FDA regulation, because FDA approval is generally required for coverage. To learn about experience in marketing emerging technologies, we focused on devices that had already been approved by the FDA.

operative care for implants, ranged up to tens of thousands of dollars.

The novelty of the emerging technologies relative to alternative therapies also ranged widely. For example, one of the devices was the second to market of two similar devices, and another involves a novel mode of action to compete with devices that are otherwise similar. Another device competes head on with a more complex and more costly device that entered the market earlier. A fourth device enables treatment of a life-threatening condition with less-invasive surgery than the standard alternative. The final technology employs a very innovative, but quite costly, approach to treating a condition for which alternative therapies are very inexpensive but often largely ineffective.

The nature and extent of available clinical evidence related to the devices also varied greatly. Most have peer-reviewed, published evidence on safety and efficacy. A few of the devices have been studied in double-blind, randomized clinical trials. However, there is no randomized evidence about some of the technologies.[5] To support claims of safety or effectiveness, some of the devices effectively piggyback on previous studies of similar devices or of a related clinical approach that has been shown to be safe or effective.[6]

In addition to clinical evidence, in today's health care environment, many purchasers, insurers, providers, and consumers want to con-

---

[5]Often, the gold standard for *clinical trials*—randomized, double-blind, placebo-controlled studies as generally used for pharmaceuticals—cannot be met for studying devices. Reasons include ethical concerns (which may prevent randomization); blinding of clinicians may be infeasible (e.g., one has to see the device to use it); and use of a placebo may be infeasible (e.g., for implantable devices, this would involve a sham operation). For discussions of the difficulty or impossibility of many device trials' meeting the gold standard and some implications, see Chang and Luft (1991, pp. 99–101), Rettig (1997, p. 51), and Ramsey et al. (1998). Ramsey et al. (1998, pp. SP190–SP191) also point to difficulties in recruiting patients to participate in clinical trials, the importance of long-term performance such as durability of implanted devices over several years, and the importance of operator skill in performing procedures (e.g., implant surgeries).

[6]Most of these studies were conducted before FDA approval. We also asked companies about studies conducted after market introduction. We were told that, typically, such studies aimed at enabling use of the device for additional indications, evaluated performance of modified designs, or focused on long-term effects or effects on populations of special concern (e.g., the elderly, patients with specific co-morbidities).

sider nonclinical issues such as costs and other economic factors in making utilization decisions.[7] A market demand for economic information is reflected in efforts by many of the companies interviewed to develop such information. The degree to which companies have invested in cost-effectiveness and economic studies—and the degree to which they have developed useful information—varied greatly over the devices discussed in the interviews. For some of the devices, there is substantial information on the overall costs of treatment or on the costs of failures to treat a condition successfully.

Who would be responsible? Some of these costs—if incurred—would be borne by MCOs or (depending on risk-sharing arrangements) providers using the technology. Other costs would be borne by patients, other insurers in the future, or society at large through taxes. Some of the costs considered by the studies are incurred within days or months of treatment; in other cases, costs that would not be incurred for several years are considered. The evidence is quite straightforward and easy to understand for some technologies; for others, the evidence is developed using complex analytic models. According to the descriptions provided by companies, adoption of some of the devices would increase costs of MCOs and would lower MCO costs for others.

RECENT EXPERIENCE IN COMMERCIALIZING DEVICES

The degree of success that the sample companies have achieved in marketing their devices to MCOs has varied widely, both across MCOs for a particular device and across devices. Some have been very successful commercially. For example, some have generally obtained positive coverage decisions when MCOs have made formal decisions, and procedures using their devices have generally been authorized whether or not there has been a formal coverage decision. For those whose success has been limited, the reasons have differed. For example, many large MCOs have approved some de-

---

[7]Sources (of varying detail and technical content) on issues and methods of economic evaluation of medical technologies are Task Force on Principles for Economic Analysis of Health Care Technology (1995), Medical Alley (1995), Gold et al. (1996), Sloan (1996), Ramsey et al. (1998), and Luce and Elixhauser (1999). The art and science of economic evaluation of medical technologies is young and is advancing rapidly.

vices for coverage, but their use has often been judged not medically necessary in individual cases. For another device, coverage has been denied or contractually excluded by many plans, but the device has been judged medically necessary in many cases by other plans. What kinds of decisions and activities by MCOs and manufacturers determine such outcomes?

Manufacturer Views on MCO Processes and Decisions

Most of the interview respondents reported that willingness of MCOs to pay for their products and associated professional services is critical to the commercial success of the devices being discussed.[8] Several respondents related that indemnity insurers were typically more willing to cover their devices and the associated professional services, and in many cases reimburse more generously. One respondent emphasized that the importance of MCOs differs substantially across the country according to the extent of market penetration by MCOs and differing degrees to which financial risk for use of the company's technology was borne by provider groups rather than by health plans. Respondents with several years of experience commercializing devices indicated that the importance of MCOs has grown enormously over the past decade or so.[9] Respondents also indicated that the importance of MCOs is growing because of the ongoing growth of managed care generally and ongoing efforts to enroll Medicare patients in managed care through the Medicare+Choice program. The latter development, of course, means that MCOs may become very important, even for devices that would be used almost exclusively by Medicare enrollees.

Manufacturers report that in their experience formal coverage reviews are infrequent.[10] Several manufacturers told us that, in their

---

[8]Recall that, for interviews, we attempted to choose companies for which this would be true.

[9]The only respondent who reported that MCO decisions were not critical to commercial success was one whose product would be used almost exclusively by Medicare-eligible patients, in which case coverage and reimbursement policies of the Medicare program were the paramount factors.

[10]For information concerning the frequency of formal coverage decisions by MCOs, see below where we report on our interviews with MCOs. Ramsey et al. (1998,

experience, various large payers undertake some formal coverage decision processes, including formal technology assessments (TAs).[11,12] In many cases, these large payers are national organizations with several affiliated health plans operating in a variety of geographic locations; however, manufacturers reported that a positive coverage decision by a national MCO does not guarantee coverage by its affiliated plans.[13]   Some manufacturers indicated that, in their experience, smaller payers rarely conduct formal coverage reviews or TAs, and many seem to follow the lead of large payers in determining their coverage policies.

Formal coverage decisions may or may not be crucial to how extensively an emerging technology is used. The manufacturers we interviewed had very different experiences in this regard. According to the manufacturers, new technologies are often reimbursed without MCO personnel even being aware of that fact. Often this situation occurs because a new technology is used by a plan's providers and billed to the plan under a pre-existing Current Procedural Terminology (CPT) code,[14] so that the bill is paid without anyone within the MCO being aware that a new technology is involved.

Delays in decisions can be costly to manufacturers and to patients. On the one hand, manufacturers whose devices were aimed at life-threatening conditions reported that, when necessary, decisions

---

p. SP191) write that, "in general, health plans focus their limited technology assessment resources on the most expensive treatments."

[11]Rettig (1997) provides a detailed description of how—and by whom—medical technology assessments are performed in the United States.

[12]Chang and Luft (1991, p. 106) report that technology assessments conducted by private insurers are often less formal and are implemented more quickly than assessments performed by government agencies (e.g., in the course of reviewing a technology for Medicare coverage) but are not necessarily less rigorous.

[13]Participants at the October 7 meeting pointed out that coverage may vary geographically among affiliated plans for several reasons, including differing state regulations or mandates, local standards of care, or litigation risks.

[14]There need not be anything deceptive about billing a new procedure under a CPT code that existed before the procedure was developed, because the description associated with the code may accurately describe the new procedure despite its being novel in some medically important way. For discussions of the use of old billing codes for new procedures and the implications of doing so, see Chang and Luft (1991, pp. 102, 104, 107), Kahn (1991, pp. 94–95), and Powe, et al. (1996). Chang and Luft (1991, p. 104) report that, if a standard code is not used, "[t]his generally requires a third-party payer to make an explicit coverage decision."

were made very expeditiously; we heard no suggestions that decision delays posed threats to life. On the other hand, some manufacturers of devices for which delays pose less danger to patients reported experiencing many instances of extensive delays—especially in formal coverage decisions. In this context, some interview respondents volunteered that MCOs had to set priorities, and that there could be very legitimate reasons for decisions about their devices to be assigned relatively low priorities.

The fact that many devices are adopted or rejected without explicit decisions by MCOs raises the question of what factors tend to attract attention by MCOs. When asked about this, manufacturers emphasized impacts of their own efforts to market their technologies to MCO medical directors—whom manufacturers uniformly described as the key decisionmakers within MCOs—and MCO case managers,[15] as well as impacts of pre-authorization requests from physicians. As we would expect, manufacturers tend to call attention to their products when they believe it is in their interest to do so—for example, when they believe that they can make a convincing case to medical directors or case managers, or because they have not been (or believe they cannot be) successful in achieving adoption without explicit decisions to cover their technologies.

We also asked manufacturers what roles they play in MCO decision processes. All stated that they provide clinical (and, sometimes, economic) information to medical directors and other MCO personnel, and to committees to be used in formal coverage reviews or case-by-case determinations of medical necessity. They also reported promoting their products and associated procedures directly to individual physicians, physician opinion leaders, medical-specialty societies, and, sometimes, directly to patients. Finally, several manufacturers reported that they help physicians and patients to document pre-authorization requests or to appeal denials.

---

[15]To contribute to both clinical and financial goals, case managers monitor and coordinate care for selected patients during illness or injury episodes. Case managers were mentioned by several of our interview respondents. Their importance was sometimes described in negative terms (i.e., they can resist pre-authorization requests and impede access to medical directors); however, because of the nature of their technologies, some manufacturers viewed case managers as natural allies, once they got their message across.

We also inquired about how MCOs use information provided to them by manufacturers. Interview respondents typically replied either that the information they provide is carefully considered or that they do not know how it is used. Manufacturers also reported that MCOs often request additional information from them, such as data about clinical effectiveness or cost-effectiveness for specific groups of patients (e.g., elderly patients, patients with specific co-morbidities, smokers). Several manufacturers also emphasized that there is enormous variation across MCOs in the information they request from manufacturers.

Of course, MCOs do not rely exclusively on information provided by manufacturers. When asked about other information used by MCOs, manufacturers typically mentioned published literature, especially if it is peer-reviewed. In addition, manufacturers reported that MCOs often obtain technology assessments from public and private organizations,[16] consider whether and under what conditions the device and associated procedures are covered by Medicare,[17] and consult with local academics or physician leaders.

---

[16]Federal agencies that conduct and publicly disseminate medical technology assessments include HCFA, AHRQ, and the National Institutes of Health (NIH). (Rettig, 1997; Ramsey et al., 1998.) Technology assessments by private organizations are generally proprietary and are made available to MCOs (and others, including hospitals, government agencies) under various financial arrangements. Rettig (1997) provides an unusually informative description of many private organizations that conduct technology assessments, including their histories, their staffing, the kinds of information they use to conduct their assessments, and services offered and their pricing. The private technology assessment organizations that were mentioned most frequently by manufacturers were ECRI, Hayes, Inc., and the Blue Cross, Blue Shield Technology Evaluation Center (BCBSA TEC), which are profiled by Rettig (1997). The National Institute for Health Care Management Research and Educational Foundation (NIHCM Foundation) (1999, pp. 17–18) also describes the procedures of the BCBSA TEC. Mendelson et al. (1995) discuss technology assessment activities of state governments.

[17]Either under national coverage policies determined by HCFA or, much more often, local coverage policies determined under quite general guidelines by the contractors that HCFA hires to process Medicare claims. "Historically, HCFA has [excluded] from Medicare coverage medical services that have not been demonstrated to be safe and effective by acceptable clinical evidence or that have not been generally accepted in the medical community as safe and effective" (General Accounting Office [GAO], 1994, Chapter 1). The National Health Policy Forum (1998, FAQs, p. 2) reports that "only about 10 to 20 treatments or technologies per year are considered by HCFA for national coverage determinations." The HCFA Coverage Issues Manual section on Durable Medical Equipment lists 17 types of durable medical equipment and 16 types of prosthetic devices (available at www.hcfa.gov/pubforms/06_cim/ci60.htm). Contractors, which include Peer Review Organizations, HMOs, commercial insurers,

Manufacturers also indicated that many MCOs are influenced by the coverage policies of other organizations. Large and small MCOs often ask manufacturers about Medicare policy regarding their technology. Manufacturers report that Medicare coverage can help them greatly in the private market and that lack of Medicare coverage can be very costly to them. Manufacturers also reported that positive coverage decisions by other private payers can help them obtain positive decisions by MCOs; indeed, manufacturers use coverage by other MCOs (that may be competitors) as a selling point. When asked for examples of private payers that appear to influence decisions of MCOs, manufacturers generally named two or three of the eight or so largest private payers in the country.

Finally, we asked manufacturers whether and how MCOs communicate their decisions to manufacturers. Most manufacturers replied that such communication is rare, and that it generally occurs only if the manufacturer expends substantial effort. For example, some manufacturers told us that they often (sometimes routinely) demand explanations for coverage denials, and that the explanations they receive tend to be brief and very carefully worded. Some manufacturers added that even when positive coverage decisions were made, medical-necessity or patient-selection criteria were often not explained to them. The most common source of manufacturer information about MCO decisions may be individual physicians who inform them of medical-necessity decisions in individual cases.

Marketing Strategies and Tactics

Commercializing new medical devices leads manufacturers to undertake a variety of tasks. Our discussions with manufacturers suggest that companies employ one of two basic strategies. The first strategy involves seeking formal coverage approvals from prominent

---

and Blue Cross/Blue Shield plans, do not have the burden of following strict technology-assessment criteria, and there are no formal checks on their compliance (Chang and Luft, 1991, pp. 105–106; see also General Accounting Office, 1994). On how HCFA decides on what technologies to review for national coverage decisions, see GAO (1994, Chapter 1): "Provided that a technology is not statutorily barred from coverage, HCFA considers several factors when deciding on the need for a national coverage decision, including the potential expense to the Medicare program, the potential for widespread use in medical practice, the level of disagreement about a technology's safety and effectiveness, and the variations among contractor coverage decisions."

MCOs and other insurers and using these approvals to influence other (e.g., small) insurers. The second strategy involves attempting to build use of the technology without explicit coverage decisions and seeking formal coverage approvals only after widespread use has been achieved—if ever.[18]

Whichever strategy is pursued, manufacturers' marketing efforts are often elaborate. The manufacturers we interviewed generally employed several of the following tactics:

- Meeting with payers and medical directors well before product launch to build awareness of the product and to solicit suggestions on how to make their informational materials more useful to decisionmakers

- Meeting with MCO medical directors after product launch to present cases for coverage and payment

- Recruiting physician champions to help gain access to medical directors and to influence specialty societies and individual physicians

- Providing professional education—for example, by disseminating information in various ways and, in some cases, by providing hands-on training in performing innovative procedures

- Attending meetings, conferences, or conventions of specialty societies, case managers, or patient groups to make their case in various ways

- Visiting individual physicians' offices to make their case

- Developing in-house staff to help physicians and patients with requests for pre-authorization and reimbursement, and appeals of coverage denials.

---

[18]Widespread use can help a manufacturer make a case for coverage, because, for example, the technology can then be claimed to have become the standard of care or because widespread physician acceptance of a technology can be viewed as evidence of safety and effectiveness.

Potential Hurdles to Device Adoption by MCOs

We usually did not ask manufacturers directly about potential impediments to MCO adoption of emerging technologies.[19] However, we gleaned considerable information of this sort from what they told us. Potential adoption hurdles should be of substantial interest to aspiring medical innovators and less-experienced device manufacturers who could benefit from a better understanding of the market environment for products they may seek to commercialize in the future. The issue should also be of substantial interest to policymakers and policy analysts who wish to consider how well these hurdles may serve the social objective of facilitating adoption of emerging technologies that deliver sufficient social value relative to costs and impeding adoption of those that do not.

Several of the manufacturers believe that they had developed convincing evidence that the emerging technologies they were marketing offered significant clinical advantages over alternative therapies. When those technologies were aimed at life-threatening conditions or serious diseases, the manufacturers generally reported being quite successful in their commercialization efforts. In contrast, if technologies were not aimed at life-threatening conditions or serious diseases, commercialization was more difficult, especially if adoption of the technology appeared to increase MCO costs in the near term, if the technology was not covered by Medicare, or both.

Some of the manufacturers told us that the advantages of their technologies over alternative therapeutic approaches included important improvements in quality of life for patients. Among these manufacturers, there appears to be general agreement that such benefits to patients are not given much weight in adoption decisions by MCOs. For example, some MCOs tended to characterize particular improvements in quality of life as improved "convenience" for patients, concluding on that basis that technologies that offered only such benefits are not medically necessary and therefore are not covered. In addition, two of the interview respondents whose devices might be characterized as contributing primarily to quality of life reported

---

[19]This issue is not directly raised in the interview protocol (Appendix B).

that their technologies were specifically excluded contractually by many MCOs or that this possibility was a serious concern to them.

Several manufacturers also averred that their commercialization efforts were inappropriately hampered by the nonpublic nature of the technology assessment, coverage decisionmaking, and medical-necessity-determination processes at most MCOs. Several of the interview respondents were concerned about the resulting restrictions on their ability to make their cases directly to committees (i.e., their written materials had to speak for themselves). Some manufacturers raised a specific concern that negative decisions may have been based on inaccurate or outdated information contained in technology assessments obtained from outside organizations to which manufacturers had no access and to which they could not offer rebuttal directly.

A hurdle faced by all manufacturers is the sheer magnitude and complexity of the tasks involved in seeking and gaining widespread market acceptance of emerging technologies:

• There are hundreds of managed care organizations in the United States, and each makes more or less independent decisions.

• MCOs have different structures and procedures for making coverage decisions.

• MCO medical directors were generally described as reasonable and dedicated to making good medical decisions; however, they are extremely busy people, and much effort is often required to gain access to them.

• Often manufacturers face the task of making large numbers of physicians aware of emerging technologies and, in some cases, training them to perform the associated procedures.[20]

---

[20]Sometimes, the relevant group is primary care physicians (PCPs). In some instances, PCPs are a key target of information-dissemination efforts, because they might use the technology themselves. In other cases, PCPs are targeted because, even though specialists would use the technology, patient referrals from PCPs often would be required.

- Finally, manufacturers face the tasks of developing clinical and economic evidence and communicating the evidence to decisionmakers.[21]

Special Hurdles for Very Innovative Technologies

Moreover, especially innovative therapies can face particularly high hurdles to adoption for any of several reasons:

- If a procedure involving a new device is quite unlike previous procedures, it may be inappropriate to use an existing CPT code, and pre-authorization or reimbursement requests are less likely to be approved without attracting attention.[22]

- When existing codes are not appropriate, the manufacturer faces the costly and time-consuming task of obtaining new codes.[23] This task generally requires showing that physicians are using the new procedure, which, in turn, requires diffusion of the technology despite the lack of appropriate CPT codes and, often, support from medical-specialty societies.[24]

- Very innovative procedures can attract mass-media attention, leading numerous patients to request or demand the new treat-

---

[21]Communicating economic evidence can be especially difficult, because medical directors, for example, are not generally well versed in economic principles or methods of cost-effectiveness analysis; in some instances, the methods and models used are necessarily complex.

[22]Use of new procedures is often recognized because of the use of unrecognized codes, absence of codes, excess charges attached to existing codes, or billing as an "unlisted procedure" with additional explanation (Chang and Luft, 1991, pp. 105–107).

[23]CPT codes are determined by American Medical Association (AMA) panels, usually based on proposals made by medical-specialty societies. During the late 1980s, there were about 7000 CPT codes; there were 500 changes in 1988 alone (Chang and Luft, 1991, p. 108).

[24]Kahn (1991, pp. 94–95) emphasizes disadvantages for a company if its technology does not fit into the existing coding system: "An innovation novel enough to be difficult to fit within the existing codes has an especially difficult acceptance by the health care system." Chang and Luft (191, p. 107) point to a potential advantage: "a new code allows for the possibility of a more generous payment." Most of our interview respondents thought it was advisable to work within the existing coding framework if possible, emphasizing that obtaining a new code is costly, a legitimate medical reason must exist, and, in any case, it is difficult to obtain premium reimbursement levels.

ment,[25] thereby raising concerns about rapid diffusion of the technology and rapid cost growth. Rapid diffusion driven by consumer demands can lead to inappropriate use. Rapid expansion of costs can be especially problematic for MCOs, because unanticipated costs are incurred before premiums can be renegotiated with payers.

- When a technology is especially innovative, the task of informing physicians can be especially daunting. In some cases, a very innovative therapy can provide the first truly effective treatment for a condition, and companies face the task of informing primary care physicians (PCPs) so that they will be more likely to refer patients to appropriate specialists. In other cases, the procedure itself may be very innovative, presenting the manufacturer with the task of providing training for physicians.

- Very innovative emerging technologies may threaten the incomes of some groups of physicians, because specialists different from those who have routinely treated the condition in the past might perform a new procedure. In such instances, the physicians who are threatened may be especially skeptical of the value of the new procedure and communicate this skepticism to MCO decisionmakers.

---

[25]Participants at the October 7 meeting added that use of the Internet can have a similar effect, which they expect will grow markedly in the years to come.

Chapter Four

HOW MCO MEDICAL DIRECTORS SEE THE SYSTEM

In this chapter, we describe and interpret our interviews with representatives of nine managed care organizations. We begin by providing background on how the managed care organizations were selected and recruited to participate, and the issues addressed in the interviews. We then report and interpret their experiences with emerging medical technologies. As with manufacturers, the discussion is somewhat general in order to avoid inadvertently revealing the identity of any participating managed care organization. Despite this limitation, we believe we convey various ways that MCOs handle emerging technologies.

BACKGROUND ON MCO INTERVIEWS

Recruitment of Interview Respondents

To understand how MCOs respond to the availability of new medical technologies, we sought to interview managed care organizations representing a substantial proportion of the managed care market in California.[1] We sought to interview a selection of organizations with

---

[1]The study focused on managed care organizations in California because of the interests of the sponsoring California Goldstrike Partnership. California is a national leader in the development and growth of managed care and has a high managed-care-penetration rate. Specifically, of Californians who receive their health insurance coverage through employers, 63 percent are enrolled in HMOs, another 23 percent receive their health care through Preferred Provider Organizations (PPOs), and only 7 percent have health care coverage through traditional indemnity insurance plans (Enthoven and Singer, 1998). The experience to date of California plans is not necessarily representative of managed care plans nationally, especially because of the high prevalence

financial responsibility and decisionmaking authority for coverage decisions, including large and medium or small MCOs and capitated medical groups contracting with MCOs.[2] To learn more about factors operating at a national level and to explore the interplay between national and local MCO decisionmaking and coverage policy, we included some plans associated with national organizations.

We identified potential MCO respondents using the 1998 California Managed Care Survey.[3] Once identified, RAND investigators contacted MCO staff to request an interview. Chief executive officers or medical directors of each MCO and capitated medical group received a letter or fax from RAND including a description of the project and its goals (Appendix A) and a description of the interview, together with a list of interview questions (Appendix C). We encouraged MCOs to use specific devices as examples in describing their processes. In particular, we asked them to think of emerging technologies for which the coverage or medical-necessity decisionmaking process had been unusually difficult.

Content of the Interviews

As detailed in Appendix C, the interviews with MCOs addressed five sets of issues:

- The extent of formal technology assessments of new medical devices, the processes employed for those assessments, and the role of manufacturers

- How the MCO makes coverage decisions for procedures involving emerging medical devices

---

in California (relative to other states) of sub-capitation contracts that put medical groups at financial risk. Nevertheless, California is an interesting case because the California market is important in and of itself.

[2]We focused on organizations that are responsible for both providing care and assuming financial risk. For a study that compares the experiences of such organizations with indemnity insurers, see Powe et al. (1996). For a study comparing reliance on technology assessment of decisionmakers in hospitals, HMOs, and third-party payers, see Luce and Brown (1995).

[3]This survey contains profiles of every significant managed care organization—including HMOs, PPOs, Medicare and Medi-Cal risk plans—operating in California, including information on statewide enrollment. The survey is published in a supplement to *California Medicine*.

- How the MCO sets payment or reimbursement levels for medical devices

- How case-by-case medical-necessity determinations are made

- Lessons learned and advice for medical device manufacturers.

Of the eleven MCOs and three capitated medical groups we approached, we were able to interview eight MCOs and one capitated medical group.[4] Typically, one respondent represented each MCO: the medical director or chief medical officer.[5] We conducted all of the interviews by telephone, and they lasted about 45 minutes each. As with the manufacturer interviews, respondents were promised confidentiality and were told they were free to decline to discuss sensitive or proprietary information. We used the questions in Appendix C as the guide and generally proceeded in the order in the protocol. As with the manufacturers, in no case did any respondent refuse to address any topic included in our protocol, nor did they seem reluctant to reveal information about their internal processes of TA and coverage decisionmaking.

Descriptions of the MCOs Interviewed

All of the MCOs we studied were based in California, although several respondents described procedures of national organizations with which they are affiliated. Respondents represented five of the ten largest MCOs in California, all with statewide enrollments of

---

[4]In our initial round of telephone calls, several MCO representatives declined to participate, and two of the three capitated medical groups we approached declined to participate, reporting that they did not do their own technology assessments. Two other studies reported in the literature employed semi-structured interviews of key decisionmakers. Weingart (1993) studied technology decisionmaking in medical centers, and Luce and Brown (1995) studied technology assessment by hospitals, HMOs, and third-party payers. Neither reported the extent of refusals to participate among potential respondents contacted. Response rates for other mail surveys, such as the survey reported in Powe et al. (1996) and in Steiner et al. (1996, 1997), are generally disappointing (e.g., 41 percent). Yet, these studies and our study include major MCOs covering the majority of health plan enrollees nationally, and in California, respectively.

[5]Other studies of technology assessment have also relied on medical directors as the key respondents. Steiner et al. (1996) report that 70 percent of respondents to their national mail survey of private health insurers were medical directors.

more than 1 million. We also interviewed medical directors of three MCOs with statewide enrollments between 75,000 and 150,000, and the medical director of one large capitated medical group. These MCOs represent a mix of for-profit and non-profit organizations, had private-sector and public-sector (e.g., Medicare, Medicaid) enrollees, and offered various insurance products (Health Maintenance Organization [HMO], Preferred Provider Organization [PPO], Medicare HMO, Medi-Cal HMO) in California.

RECENT MCO EXPERIENCES WITH TECHNOLOGY ADOPTION

MCOs described a multilayered process of decisionmaking that results in a procedure,[6] and any devices involved, becoming eligible for payment or reimbursement. According to the MCO respondents, decisions about technology adoption involve interpretation of contract language ("business" decisions), as well as assessment of whether the medical procedure represents the standard of care ("medical" decisions). A threshold question for the MCO is, "Does the payer's contract specifically exclude the procedure or device?"[7] If the medical procedure or the device is specifically excluded, there may be no need for further review.[8] If the procedure is not specifically excluded by the payer's contract, the MCO then needs to make a decision about whether to pay for use of the procedure. This process is generally referred to by MCOs as *coverage decisionmaking.*

To make a coverage decision, MCOs often employ technology assessment to evaluate the properties of a medical technology, assessing the safety, effectiveness, and indications for that technology's use. Technology assessments may be formal, involving various staff

---

[6]MCOs reported that they evaluate medical procedures and not devices per se. In reviewing a medical procedure, they consider evidence about any device or devices used in the treatment.

[7]The contract between the payer (typically an employer) and the managed care organization articulates the rights and responsibilities and the flow of funds and assignment of financial risk. Most important in this context, it defines the covered health benefits.

[8]Payers' contracts determine what services will be covered, unless the contract appears to be in conflict with a government mandate or there are concerns about possible litigation if coverage is denied. See, for example, Havighurst (1995).

and one or more committees, or they may be informal, performed, for example, entirely by the MCO medical director.[9] Coverage decisions are based on the evidence incorporated in the technology assessment and on contract interpretation. These decisions determine whether a procedure is experimental or investigational or represents the standard of care. A positive decision on coverage does not mean that every enrollee has access to the procedure, however. If a positive coverage decision is made, MCOs have processes for determining whether the procedure is medically necessary in particular cases.

Triggers for Formal Coverage Decisionmaking

Our MCO respondents reported that they generally lack systematic surveillance mechanisms for new technologies, which makes them reactive rather than proactive. They tend to react to triggers such as physician and patient demand, prior-authorization requests, and claims submitted without a CPT code.[10] MCOs report being influenced by their competitors only indirectly. Specifically, when several of their physicians report receiving payment from one of their competitors, an MCO is likely to assess whether it should cover the procedure. Whether a procedure is considered for a formal technology assessment depends on the number and pattern of requests. A large number of requests, several requests from a particular provider (indicating that a new device is being tried), or even a single request may trigger a technology assessment.[11] Owing to time and staffing

---

[9]As described in Chapter Three, new technologies often are introduced into managed care systems largely without the knowledge of MCOs and without any conscious decisions about adoption. This "under-the-radar" phenomenon has been described in other studies; for example, Powe et al. (1996) report that health care plans were often not aware that a physician was using a new technology if it was billed using a standard billing code. In this chapter, we report on MCO experiences in making explicit decisions about technology adoption.

[10]From a national survey of health plans, Powe et al. (1996) report that provider queries (85 percent), higher-than-usual charges (57 percent), utilization review activities (48 percent), and patient queries (33 percent) were the most frequently cited factors alerting health plans to the use of new laser technologies.

[11]Single requests tend to trigger technology assessments only when the MCO believes that the procedure may be experimental or investigational. Similarly, Powe et al. (1996) report that the single-most-important clinical factor prompting medical directors of health plans to make a specific coverage decision on laser angioplasty technology was the belief on the part of the medical director that the procedure might be

constraints, not all procedures are given a formal review; however, all MCOs have processes for making coverage decisions in the absence of a formal technology assessment.

The Technology Assessment Processes of MCOs

The formal technology assessment process varies widely across MCOs, according to our respondents.[12] Aspects that vary include the following:

- The level of formality, including whether the MCO uses staff in addition to the medical director and one or more standing committees to conduct the technology assessment[13]

- The level of responsibility for decisionmaking—for example, whether the decisions are made by the national headquarters or by the local health plans

- The rigor—depth and breadth—of the review of medical evidence[14]

---

experimental. Other important clinical factors include complication rates and questions about whether the technology reflected standard practice in the community.

[12]For detailed descriptions of formal technology-assessment processes, see Braslow et al. (1998) describing United HealthCare's TA process and Parrish (1998) describing the TA process used by Blue Shield of California. NIHCM Foundation (1999, pp. 11–13) provides less-detailed descriptions of the coverage decision processes of Highmark Blue Cross Blue Shield, and Blue Cross of California.

[13]The medical director is a key participant in the process of technology assessment in all of the MCOs interviewed for our study. However, there was great variability in the number and types of additional staff and committees involved in the process. Some MCOs have multiple layers of review. Steiner et al. (1996) reported that 92 percent of respondents in their national mail survey indicated that the medical director was directly involved in the review process. Forty-six percent indicated that it was left to the medical director's discretion to decide when to refer the decision to a committee or another staff member in the health plan.

[14]MCOs rely on a variety of sources of information, including, but not limited to, journal articles retrieved through Medline searches, government-agency (FDA, HCFA, and AHRQ) materials, information supplied by manufacturers, TAs performed by other insurers, and opinions of national and local experts. Similarly, Steiner et al. (1996) report that the most frequently ranked sources of information used by health plans are medical journals, opinions of local experts, FDA clearance documents, and information from plan associations such as Blue Cross and Blue Shield.

- The use of outside expertise and resources, including technology-assessment organizations such as ECRI and Hayes, Inc., and national or local physician experts

- The extent to which MCOs are influenced by government agencies, such as AHRQ (formerly AHCPR) and HCFA, and health insurance industry leaders

- The average number of formal technology reviews conducted each year.[15]

Some aspects of the technology assessment processes are common across MCOs. Typically, for example, FDA approval of the medical device involved in the procedure is necessary before a technology assessment will be performed. FDA approval is considered by all MCOs to be necessary but not sufficient for their purposes.[16] All MCO respondents also reported that their staff conduct literature searches using the National Library of Medicine's Medline search engine, and gather other information, including information from the manufacturers. The medical director and other MCO staff then weigh the strength of the evidence, although some MCOs employ more-systematic procedures than others do. MCO respondents report using outside sources most often when a Medline search produces conflicting information or when the decision is especially difficult.[17]

Participation of Manufacturers in the TA Process

Most formal TA processes are "closed": Manufacturers may submit written materials but are not allowed to participate directly in the

---

[15]There was a wide range in reported numbers of formal technology assessments per year. Most MCOs reported between three and 15, with one MCO reporting 36.

[16]Several MCO respondents noted that the FDA reviews devices with a focus on safety, and to some extent efficacy (effects under clinical trial conditions), but not effectiveness (under routine clinical practice conditions) or cost-effectiveness. Thus, they believe FDA approval is only a starting point. They report, with a sense of frustration, that many manufacturers seem perplexed by their unwillingness to accept FDA approval as sufficient for coverage.

[17]For example, when procedures are in the process of evolving from being considered experimental to representing the standard of care or standard practice in that community.

decisionmaking process. Of the nine MCOs we interviewed, only two reported that manufacturers were invited, at least on occasion, to participate in the TA committee process.

MCO respondents also characterized the information provided by manufacturers. On the one hand, most MCO respondents viewed information provided by manufacturers as a "useful starting point." Several expressed the general attitude that, "if they have information, we'd love to see it." On the other hand, many of the MCO respondents regarded literature reviews produced by manufacturers somewhat skeptically. Respondents noted that manufacturers usually did not report the keywords used in computer-aided literature searches, making it difficult for MCOs to assess the quality of the literature review. MCO respondents generally expressed concern that manufacturers tend to include studies that support their position and ignore evidence that might undermine their arguments. Medical directors stated that they accord the same weight to manufacturer-supported, peer-reviewed studies as to other such studies, but review the design and methodology especially carefully.[18]

Most MCO respondents expressed a desire for less marketing on the part of the manufacturers. Most medical directors did not believe that the technology-assessment process was an appropriate forum for a sales pitch. One medical director summed it up this way: "The harder they push, the more resistance they'll get."[19]

Nonmedical Factors Affecting Coverage Decisions

MCOs also consider nonmedical factors in making coverage decisions. Nonmedical factors considered by our MCO respondents include the following:

---

[18]Similarly, participants in a recent symposium expressed the view that, if scientific evidence comes solely from "advocates" (such as manufacturers), "it is critical to evaluate the validity of the evidence, including whether the studies conform to FDA regulations" (NIHCM Foundation, 1999, p.32).

[19]One MCO respondent said that he and his colleagues prefer "permission marketing," which he described as "letting the device speak for itself." He suggested that manufacturers allow MCOs to get some experience with the device and wait for MCOs to approach them for information—in effect, inviting the manufacturer to market the product then.

- state insurance mandates and other state regulatory requirements

- publicity about and controversy surrounding a procedure or medical device

- demand for a technology among patients and physicians

- competition with other health plans[20]

- potential for litigation.[21]

Generally, MCO medical directors suggest that medical factors—evidence from the technology assessment—carry the greatest weight in decisionmaking, but that nonmedical factors can also be important, especially publicity or controversy that may result in a high level of demand from patients and physicians, including some demand viewed as inappropriate by some medical directors.[22]

Reconsideration of Coverage Decisions

Negative coverage decisions are sometimes reconsidered if important new data emerge, if there is continued physician or patient demand, or if the MCO decides that covering an emerging technology would confer a market advantage. In addition, some regulatory and accreditation bodies require periodic reconsideration. Medical directors do not routinely report negative coverage decisions to manufacturers, and no medical director suggested that manufacturers have any effect on whether they reconsider a coverage decision.

---

[20]One MCO respondent, reflecting on the issue of competition, said, "We don't want to get out too far ahead but we don't want to lag too far behind either."

[21]MCOs want to use processes that will result in fair decisions that can be supported in the face of litigation. Documentation of decisionmaking is critical in the litigation context.

[22]Powe et al. (1996) also report on the importance of nonmedical factors in coverage decisionmaking. The nonclinical factors most often cited by their health plan survey respondents included high potential cost (36 percent), possible liability risk (15 percent), and the percentage of the insured population that would be affected (13 percent).

Determining Payment Levels for New Devices

After making a coverage decision (whether that decision is based on a formal technology assessment or on a more informal process), the MCO must set a payment level. Medical directors reported that they are not directly involved in determining payment rates, but stated that payment levels generally reflect market forces. Pricing is often based on the existence and price of alternatives and on the projected use of the product. With new devices, the MCO may price based on a similar product. For very novel devices, which are more difficult to price, the MCO may use Medicare reimbursement rates or attempt to negotiate with the manufacturer on the basis of volume.[23]

Case-by-Case Determinations of Medical Necessity

MCO respondents reported that they typically develop patient-selection criteria and disseminate medical indications for procedures that have received coverage approval. These materials usually are disseminated either electronically or on paper to their physicians and physician groups. Most MCOs make case-by-case medical-necessity determinations locally, even if coverage decisions are made nationally.[24] MCOs that provide care through contracts with capitated medical groups may delegate medical-necessity decisions to them.[25]

---

[23]Powe et al. (1996) concluded that some health plans may attempt to use payment policy rather than coverage policy to control the use of emerging medical technology. They warn that such an approach could result in lower-cost, but less-effective, technologies proliferating at the expense of more-costly, but more-effective, alternatives.

[24]There is substantial confusion and disagreement about the meaning of the term "medical necessity." (For example, NIHCM Foundation, 1999, pp. 25–29.) We did not provide a definition of "medical necessity" to respondents, and none asked for a definition. Apparently, the term is not ambiguous to any of the medical directors we interviewed, although we did not explore how much disagreement there might be among them.

[25]Because capitated medical groups bear the financial risk by accepting a flat fee to provide covered benefits to a specific group of individuals, MCOs are not at risk for the costs of specific procedures and may therefore delegate the decisionmaking to the medical group, which has assumed the risk. Some of our respondents noted that tensions can arise between the health plan and the medical group when, for example, a patient successfully appeals a coverage denial by the medical group to the health plan, and the medical group bears the financial cost. This concern was also raised in the symposium summarized in NIHCM (1999, p. 14).

Medical directors report that these decisions can be especially difficult when the patient or the physician argues on what MCOs view as "nonmedical" grounds. Some MCO respondents referred to arguments made on nonmedical grounds as "quality-of-life" arguments and others referred to them as "convenience" arguments.[26] Some participants at the October 7 meeting expressed confusion about the distinction between *quality of life* and *convenience* and suggested that some MCO decisionmakers characterize some advantages for patients as "nonmedical" when, in fact, they involve genuine medical concerns.[27]

Denials of coverage can also be difficult in cases of life-threatening illnesses. In all cases, patients have the right of appeal for denial of coverage. In California, if the procedure has to do with a life-threatening condition, patients have special rights.[28] At least one MCO reported that if the procedure is requested for a patient with a terminal condition, the MCO automatically sends the patient's appeal for external review. Terminal conditions pose especially difficult situations for MCOs, because decisions must often be made very quickly.

---

[26]One MCO medical director used the example of an insulin pump, arguing that a diabetic patient may want the pump for its greater convenience, even though his or her condition was controlled with injectable insulin. The MCO would be under pressure in that situation to approve the use, even though the device was not believed to be medically necessary.

[27]Braslow et al. (1998) discuss the need to assess the "medical appropriateness" of the procedure as a part of the TA process. They define *medical appropriateness* as ensuring that "the expected health benefits from a medical service are *clinically significant* and exceed health risks by a sufficiently wide margin so that the service is demonstrably worthwhile and superior to other services (including no service)." They define *clinical significance* as including such outcomes as increased life expectancy, improved functional capacity, prevention of complications, or relief of pain. If one accepts this definition of clinical significance, one might argue that these outcomes are clearly medical outcomes; yet, it could be argued that the relief of pain could also be considered a quality-of-life outcome. We are unaware of any clear, widely accepted distinctions between medical and nonmedical outcomes or between convenience and quality of life.

[28]*California Health and Safety Code*, § 1370.4 (1997).

Chapter Five

ADVICE FOR MANUFACTURERS

ADVICE FROM EXPERIENCED MANUFACTURERS TO ASPIRING MANUFACTURERS

Part of the second goal of the project was to develop information that could help organizations hoping to develop and commercialize medical devices to understand the managed care market environment and to prepare accordingly. We asked interview respondents representing manufacturers to offer advice for such organizations. Interview respondents generally offered extensive and thoughtful answers to this query. While emphases differed across interviews, some consistent messages emerged. We first summarize advice that was offered—in one form or another—in most (and in some cases, virtually all) of our interviews with manufacturers. We then briefly relate advice that was offered by a minority of the respondents.

Almost all of the interview respondents emphasized early development of commercialization strategies and planning of commercialization efforts. One especially experienced respondent emphasized that a strategy should be developed when the "product is just an idea"—that it was not good business practice to put effort into developing a new device unless there was reason to believe that a viable commercialization strategy could be developed and implemented.[1]

---

[1]In contrast, a participant in the October 7 meeting took exception to this advice, saying, "If the technology is good enough, you have to throw your heart in before your head."

Despite lack of agreement about precisely when companies should begin to prepare for commercialization, virtually all manufacturers emphasized that companies should analyze several issues well before a product is ready for FDA review, including the following:

- Prevalence, incidence, and patient demographics of the disease or medical condition at which the product is aimed. Such information is critical to understanding the potential size of the market and who the key payers will be.

- Effectiveness, safety, and costs of existing alternatives to the product. These factors determine the nature of the competition that the new product will face. To be successful in the marketplace, a new product generally will need to demonstrate superiority to alternatives on at least one of these dimensions.

- Availability and levels of reimbursement for similar devices. The current reimbursement environment for devices similar to the one under development can provide the best guide to the situation the new device will face. Several respondents cautioned that it is very difficult to command a premium price in today's marketplace—even if a device has superior performance—and that the current reimbursement situation might reasonably be interpreted as a realistic or even optimistic projection of what the future will hold.[2,3]

- Reimbursement codes and reimbursement levels for professional and institutional services associated with the device. Several respondents emphasized that these factors can be critical, for example, to the enthusiasm of physicians and hospitals for performing or scheduling procedures that use the device.

---

[2]At least one participant at the October 7 meeting expressed the opinion that many manufacturers lack a fundamental understanding of the payment system, including coding issues and who is at risk for what dollars.

[3]When we asked how companies might project potential reimbursement levels for devices with no similar predecessors, a few respondents suggested that reimbursement levels would have to reflect demonstrated product value. Others merely indicated that projecting is *much* harder in that situation. These rather unspecific comments may, in fact, be the most useful general advice that can be offered, because it seems likely that the best approaches to projecting reimbursement for very innovative devices will typically be context-specific.

- Importance of Medicare coverage. Depending on patient demographics, use of the product by or on behalf of Medicare patients can be crucial to commercial success. If so, it is critical to understand the procedures for seeking national Medicare coverage from the HCFA. And, because national coverage decisions are made fairly infrequently, it is perhaps more important to understand the coverage policies of the numerous Medicare contractors that process claims for the HCFA.[4]

Almost all interview respondents emphasized early planning of clinical and economic studies. In this regard, respondents suggested the following:

- When planning studies, ask payers what kind of information they would find useful in making coverage and medical-necessity decisions. Several interview respondents indicated that, in their experience, payers are willing to play this role.

- Develop clear, evidence-based guidelines for appropriate use. This information can be critical in determining FDA-approved indications, which determine the claims that companies may make in marketing. Moreover, this information can be very helpful to MCOs in developing patient-selection criteria for medical-necessity determinations and can help allay concerns about inappropriate use and rapidly expanding costs.

- Design studies to do more than is typically required for FDA approval. Specifically, compare the new device to alternatives in terms of safety, efficacy, and cost. One interview respondent emphasized that, because a new technology must compete with the standard of care, companies should develop evidence about its technology relative to the current standard of care, as well as to other approaches that could become the standard by the time the new device is ready for market.

- Work with centers of excellence in designing and executing studies. High-quality studies published in highly respected,

---

[4]Such as local "fiscal intermediaries" and "carriers," and regional "durable medical equipment carriers" (National Health Policy Forum, 1998, pp. 3–4).

peer-reviewed journals can be enormously valuable in commercialization efforts.

- Involve potential physician champions—national or regional opinion leaders—in studies. Physician champions can be very helpful in influencing other physicians, in easing access to medical directors, and in making a case to medical societies.

- Make sure, however, that any studies that are undertaken are good investments. Studies cost money, and they take time. Extra time spent doing studies can delay product introduction and the generation of revenue, thereby threatening the financial viability of the product.

Finally, one or two interview respondents offered the following pieces of advice that seem well worth considering: (1) try to work within the existing coding system; (2) ground your marketing program on evidence that you expect to be able to develop; (3) earn the trust of medical directors; (4) plan to build momentum and involve specialty societies; and (5) create an in-house team to support early adopters.

ADVICE FROM MCOs TO MANUFACTURERS

Almost all of the MCO medical directors emphasized that manufacturers should make their clinical studies as rigorous as possible and accept that FDA approval is not sufficient to warrant coverage of a device. MCO respondents warn manufacturers not to push products that lack substantial clinical evidence, because they will not receive approval and will create suspicion about the manufacturer in its future dealings with the MCO.

MCOs also offered advice about marketing strategies and tactics. Because most of the MCO contracts with payers are annual or multi-year contracts, it can be very difficult for MCOs to accommodate expensive devices without warning. Medical directors recommend strongly that manufacturers not "drop devices on the market" without prior information-sharing with MCOs. The creation of an "early-warning system" was desired. The MCO medical directors were unanimous in expressing irritation about direct marketing of devices to patients and physicians. While they acknowledge that MCOs do respond to patient and physician demand, they also point out that floods of requests may cause heightened concern about inappropriate use. Specifically, MCOs need time to complete their technology-assessment processes, and high demand arising over a short time period tends to short-circuit that process. MCOs also suggest the development and implementation of a standard format for manufacturers to present information to MCOs, including the specification of medical-evidence selection criteria (such as Medline search terms).

In general, the MCOs were not entirely satisfied with the current processes of technology adoption, but there was no consensus on strategies that might be employed by MCOs and manufacturers to improve these processes. MCO medical directors differed widely in their enthusiasm for engaging in joint efforts with manufacturers.

At least one MCO medical director offered each of the following suggestions, although none was endorsed by all:

- Manufacturers should help MCOs anticipate what is "in the pipeline" and the potential costs for new technologies.

- Manufacturers should share information on experience with medical devices across MCOs and providers.

- Manufacturers and MCOs should foster cooperative clinical research—for example, manufacturers would supply the devices at a reduced cost to give the MCO and its providers some experience with the device in routine clinical settings.

- Manufacturers and MCOs should facilitate cooperative provider education—for example, by creating programs for training surgeons in the implantation of devices—in order to reduce complications and improve quality of care.

- Manufacturers and MCOs should create purchasing contracts that enable MCOs to obtain upgraded versions of expensive, multi-use devices—for example, new diagnostic imaging equipment—at reduced cost as improvements are made.

- MCOs should allow manufacturers to participate in an open technology-assessment process or to recommend physicians who are experienced with their devices.

A general lesson from the interviews is that the issue of technology adoption is a much higher priority for the manufacturers than for medical directors of California MCOs, and a much higher priority for some MCOs than for others. It is hardly surprising that MCO medical directors are not as focused on technology adoption as are manufacturers: New technologies are the lifeblood of the manufacturers we interviewed. It is unclear whether MCO personnel other than medical directors, such as those involved in marketing or in contracting with payers, are more focused on technology-adoption issues than are medical directors.

Chapter Six

HOW MIGHT TECHNOLOGY ADOPTION BE IMPROVED?

We conducted in-depth interviews with eight medical device manu-facturers and nine managed care organizations about the processes of technology assessment and technology adoption by MCOs. Combining information from these interviews, the discussion at the October 7 meeting, and the literature provides an incomplete, yet in many ways revealing, view of these processes. This view, in turn, suggests several issues that might be confronted in hopes of improv-ing the system.

BALANCING COSTS AND BENEFITS OF TECHNOLOGY ADOPTION

No matter how much society values medical care and medical inno-vation, it must also accept the relevance of costs of delivering health care under private insurance arrangements.[1] While medical innova-tion is believed to be a leading cause of increasing costs of medical care, the consequent improvements in health are highly valued by consumers.[2] Undoubtedly, some medical innovations that are

---

[1]Organizations insuring and delivering health care cannot long survive in the mar-ketplace without covering their costs. Payers and consumers care very much about how much they pay for care, both directly and indirectly, through insurance premi-ums. Premium levels are an important cause of lack of health insurance by many Americans.

[2]Newhouse (1993, p. 163) argues that the most plausible explanation for the bulk of increases in medical care costs over time has been technological advance in medicine. He emphasizes, however, that the key questions are whether the well-being of con-

adopted improve consumer well-being and others do not. In principle, comparing the social benefits and costs of medical care for individual technologies is the best way of promoting consumer well-being through medical-technology adoption.

Stated generally, we as a society should want medical technologies—new or old—to be used in particular circumstances if and only if the social benefits of use exceed the social costs.[3] Moreover, it seems safe to presume that doing a better job of implementing this criterion would also provide socially appropriate incentives for inventors, innovators, and investors.[4]

Striking an appropriate balance between benefits and costs is very difficult, and the stakes are high. Use of unproven technologies involves risks of injuries to patients, lost patient benefits from failing to use a different technology, and wasted resources. But, of course, all successful technologies were initially unproven, and limiting or delaying use of new technologies also involves risks: lost benefits to patients who could have been treated more effectively, and taking the profit out of innovation, thus reducing incentives to innovate,[5] among others.

---

sumers is improved by particular innovations, despite their costs, and states that such "questions [are] exceedingly difficult to answer."

[3] *Social benefits of medical care* include all of the consequences that improve the well-being of patients over their lifetimes—including increased length of life, reduced morbidity, improved functioning, lessened pain, any other beneficial effects—and benefits to any members of society in the form of social costs avoided (e.g., lost productivity, future treatment or rehabilitation costs) because the care is provided. *Social costs of medical care* include the value of all resources required to make decisions about and deliver the care, no matter who bears these costs (e.g., payers, insurers, providers, patients).

[4] If inventors and innovators believe that demand for their products will be higher the greater the social benefits their products can deliver, this will provide strong incentives to focus their efforts on research and development aimed at technologies satisfying the benefit-cost criterion.

[5] Ramsey et al. (1998, p. SP192) discuss the trade-off between adopting technologies more and less rapidly. Sheingold (1998, p. SP123) emphasizes risks of adopting too quickly. Eisenberg (1999, p. 1867) writes: "The worst-case scenario could be a restriction on coverage to those services for which there is evidence of effectiveness, but no resources being spent on obtaining the evidence.... Policymakers need to remember that the absence of evidence of effectiveness is not the same as evidence of the absence of effectiveness."

The enormous complexity of the processes determining such consequences and the substantial uncertainty about most elements of the calculus mean that coming close to perfection in winnowing technologies is not possible. The social goal should be identifying and implementing means of getting closer to the ideal.

MCOs AND THE TECHNOLOGY-ADOPTION PROCESS

Amid all this complexity and uncertainty, managed care organizations make decisions that can have crucial effects on medical-technology adoption and innovation. MCOs influence technology adoption by performing two broad functions: (1) determining, along with payers, the contractual contexts in which care will be organized, delivered, and financed; and (2) undertaking various activities, including contracting with providers, developing coverage policies, determining how much to pay providers or reimburse patients when care is delivered, and instituting procedures for managing care, such as practice guidelines and pre-authorization and other forms of utilization review.

However, it is essential to recognize that technology adoption is also greatly affected by factors beyond the control of MCOs. As a practical matter, for example, MCOs cannot completely control behavior of their providers and enrollees that can have profound effects on technology adoption. Technology adoption also depends on coverage and payment policies of public insurance programs (e.g., Medicare, Medicaid), preferences of private payers (expressed in contract negotiations), government mandates that constrain MCO behavior, litigation exposure, government support for medical research and technology assessment, and the behavior of manufacturers.

Our interviews with both MCOs and manufacturers and review of the existing literature indicate that, in many cases, careful and critical consideration of clinical evidence may play little or no role in technology adoption. In particular, technologies are often adopted by individual physicians and paid for by MCOs without any conscious decisions or oversight by MCOs. Technologies adopted through this route are unlikely to have been evaluated in cost-benefit terms: As a rule, physicians are not in a position to carefully and capably consider, evaluate, and weigh the relevant clinical evidence before making adoption decisions.[6,7]

Our interviews and the literature also suggest that some technologies, including especially costly or novel technologies, are subjected to substantial scrutiny by MCOs. Our interviews with MCOs suggest—and participants in the October 7 meeting generally agreed—that the available clinical evidence about an emerging technology is often equivocal, and that coverage and medical-necessity decisions often require considerable guesswork and judgment. It is unclear how well the tension between adopting too quickly or too slowly is currently being resolved. Even assuming for the sake of argument that MCOs have strong incentives to adopt new technologies slowly in order to limit costs,[8] government mandates and threats of litigation can push in the opposite direction.

IMPROVING CLINICAL INFORMATION

A major difficulty in making appropriate decisions about adopting emerging technologies is limited information about the performance of these technologies, both absolutely and in comparison with alternative technologies. This issue seems to get the most attention in the literature and in practice. We consider it at some length presently, followed by brief discussions of several other seemingly important challenges in improving the processes of technology adoption by MCOs.

What are the prospects for improving the clinical information available to MCOs for making technology-adoption decisions? It is helpful to distinguish four elements of information availability.

---

[6]See, for example, Grimes (1993).

[7]Little solace is provided by recognizing that many technologies that are adopted without much awareness or concern by MCOs are sufficiently similar to established technologies to be reimbursed under existing codes, and thus are likely in many cases to be similar to technologies already in use, because many of these earlier technologies were themselves not adopted on the basis of careful weighing of evidence.

[8]According to our interviews with MCO medical directors, costs play a role primarily in the negotiation of contracts with payers.

- **Developing better information before market introduction.**
  Some of our interview respondents, participants in the October 7
  meeting, and some commentators apparently believe that many
  device trials could have been designed, implemented, and reported to deliver more useful information with little or no increase in cost.[9] In contrast, increasing the sizes of clinical trials
  (numbers of patients) would typically involve higher costs.
  Increasing costs of clinical trials or delaying market introduction
  of promising technologies can threaten the financial viability of
  socially worthwhile innovation efforts.

- **Learning more from experience in the marketplace.** Often,
  there is much to be learned about the safety, effectiveness, and
  costs of new technologies after they enter the marketplace. Even
  the highest-quality and most extensive clinical trials leave much
  unknown.[10] Our interviews, the October 7 meeting, and the literature suggest that there is marked interest in finding ways for
  MCOs and manufacturers to work together to introduce technologies into the marketplace using approaches that would allow
  more to be learned from experience. This process might involve,
  for example, collecting systematic information on outcomes,
  creating mechanisms to pool such information, and, in some
  cases, initially restricting use of new technologies to physicians
  or facilities that are expected to have the best results.[11]

---

[9]Ramsey et al. (1998, pp. SP198–SP199) suggest guidelines—developed by the Task
Force on Technology Assessment of Medical Devices—for technology assessment of
therapeutic medical devices. Rettig (1997, p. 106) discusses the view that clinical trials
are often not well designed to provide useful information to those making decisions
about whether and how technologies will be used in routine clinical practice.

[10]Clinical trials illuminate efficacy or performance of the technology when applied by
experts. How well a technology will perform under routine clinical (i.e., less favorable)
conditions can be established only from broader use. Moreover, unlike drugs, devices
are often modified after market introduction, in attempts to improve performance
(Ramsey et al., 1998, p. SP191).

[11]Buto (1994) and Adler (1996) discuss such possibilities in the context of Medicare
and private insurance, respectively. See also Eisenberg (1999, pp. 1867–1868) and
NIHCM Foundation (1999, p. 32). Along these lines, in December 1999 health insurers
in New Jersey agreed to cover the costs of routine care for their enrollees who
participate in clinical trials for cancer therapies. The research sponsors would still be
responsible for covering the administrative costs of the trials and the drugs under
study (Kolata and Eichenwald, 1999).

- **Evaluating and synthesizing clinical information.** Technology-assessment functions are performed by many public and private organizations. Government agencies perform technology assessments and sponsor others; these assessments are generally available to the public. Many larger private insurers and MCOs perform in-house evaluations to support internal decisionmaking, and other private organizations perform technology assessments for insurers, MCOs, and government agencies. Many privately produced technology assessments are proprietary. Little is known about the general quality of these assessments, which undoubtedly varies over organizations and particular cases.[12] While it can be difficult for manufacturers to be objective about their own technologies, they are knowledgeable about them and the existence of evidence. The feasibility, advantages, and disadvantages of allowing manufacturers to comment on proprietary assessments—as part of the MCO technology assessment or coverage-decisionmaking process—is worth exploring. The extent to which purchasers of assessments detect and the market rewards higher-quality assessment will affect the general state of technology adoption.

- **Disseminating information.** Two methods for improving dissemination of information[13] are standardizing forms for reporting and improving communication between insurers and manufacturers.[14] The activities of the private technology-assessment industry, which seems to be growing in importance, expand the scope of technology assessment, and reduce—relative to complete decentralization—social costs from duplicative efforts. However, private organizations must cover their costs and, therefore, cannot be economically viable without restricting access to their reports. How this industry evolves will

---

[12]Sheingold (1998, pp. SP122–SP123) comments on duplication of effort across technology assessors and the uneven quality of assessments. Some manufacturers reported in interviews that proprietary assessments can be of poor quality or out of date.

[13]Ramsey et al. (1998, p. SP192) point to some factors limiting availability of existing information.

[14]For example, Ramsey et al. (1998, pp. SP196–SP197) propose guidelines for information exchange between manufacturers and insurers.

determine the extent to which it promotes socially beneficial technology adoption in the future.[15]

OTHER ISSUES THAT WARRANT CONSIDERATION

Our interviews, discussion at the October 7 meeting, and literature suggest other important issues that affect the quality of technology adoption.

Aligning Private Incentives of MCOs and Payers with Social Values

MCO decisions about technology adoption are made within a context determined by contract negotiations with payers. The cost-conscious, competitive environments in which MCOs market their products limit greatly the extent to which they can factor into their decisions social costs they do not bear or social benefits for which they cannot capture revenues. Our interviews suggest examples: (1) reduced treatment costs years down the road when these savings are unlikely to accrue to the MCO bearing the current treatment costs; and (2) treatment benefits that are of significant value to consumers but that might reasonably be characterized as "nonmedical."

Expecting or imploring MCOs or payers to act substantially in conflict with their self-interest[16] is not realistic, especially given the state of competition among health plans and pressures from payers to limit premium increases. Better information for employees and consumers about the quality of care delivered by different MCOs could help, but developing and implementing quality reporting systems that could effectively discipline the market to make socially appropriate adoption decisions about individual technologies is not plausible any time soon. Perhaps the best hope is more government tar-

---

[15]For example, a consolidation of the TA industry or expanding demand for TA industry services might lead to lower prices for proprietary technology assessments (since almost all costs of assessment are fixed), wider dissemination of particular assessments, assessment of more technologies, and reduced duplication of effort.

[16]For example, the Guidelines for Technology Assessment of Therapeutic Medical Devices include: "Conducting the analysis from a societal viewpoint or perspective is strongly encouraged" (Ramsey et al., 1998, p. SP199).

geting of funding for basic and clinical research related to medical technologies that provide delayed health benefits or other social benefits to which the market may fail to give adequate weight.

Enhancing MCO Capabilities to Evaluate Technologies and Make Decisions

The most obvious possible steps in this direction, such as devoting more resources to technology assessment and coverage decision-making, are appropriately left to individual MCOs to consider. However, there may be a role for collective action in providing training in technology-assessment methods or general information to MCOs. Regarding the latter, it may be helpful to provide MCOs with information about, for example, what FDA approval of devices and Medicare coverage of technologies do and do not imply about safety, effectiveness, and costs of emerging technologies.[17]

Improving Decisions by Physicians

Our interviews, the discussion at the October 7 meeting, and the literature provide an ample basis to conclude that, in many cases, technology adoption for managed care enrollees is being driven by decisions of individual physicians, not of MCOs. This is unlikely to change any time soon. Improving physician decisions—e.g., by wider development, dissemination, and use of practice guidelines or information systems—might greatly improve the technology-adoption process. Providing physicians with information about FDA regulation of devices and development of Medicare-coverage policies might also be beneficial.

---

[17]In the case of the FDA, our respondents and the literature suggest that many MCO decisionmakers are not familiar with the varying degrees to which devices are scrutinized before they are approved for marketing. For example, "many purchasers and providers are unaware that clinical testing and regulation of medical devices is vastly different from that for pharmaceutical products" (Ramsey, 1998, p. SP188). In the case of Medicare, many MCO decisionmakers may not be aware of how infrequently the HCFA makes national coverage decisions, how long these decisions generally take, and the extent to which technologies are reviewed by Medicare contractors before they are accepted or rejected for coverage.

Reducing Use of Inappropriate or Obsolete Technologies

The substantial attention to technology *adoption* tends to deflect attention from another important social objective: reducing use of technologies that are dangerous, do not work in many or all of the circumstances in which they are used, or for which superior alternatives are available.[18]

Reducing Costs of Decisionmaking for Manufacturers and MCOs

Manufacturer interview respondents pointed to the high costs of attempting to make their cases to numerous insurers. Mainly because of time and money costs, MCOs review and make formal coverage decisions about a small fraction of new technologies. Some standardizing of procedures for developing and exchanging information could be helpful.[19]

Improving Manufacturer Understanding of the Market Environment

Our interviews with manufacturers and MCOs and the discussion at the October 7 meeting suggest that some device developers and manufacturers, especially inexperienced ones, have very limited understanding of the managed care market environment. Such misunderstandings can lead innovators and manufacturers to fail financially. When their efforts are misguided, society loses as well: resources are wasted, and opportunities may be lost to develop commercially successful and medically beneficial technologies. In our interviews we have collected—and reported above—advice from both manufacturers and MCOs that could help medical innovators better anticipate the market environments they will face. However, this advice pertains to the environment as it exists today. U.S. health care organization and financing are in a state of flux; major changes are

---

[18]For example, Rettig (1997, p. 104) reports that technology assessors pay almost no attention to obsolete technologies.

[19]For example, along the lines of the guidelines proposed by the Task Force on Technology Assessment of Medical Devices (Ramsey et al., 1998).

likely because of market forces and changes in regulatory and public reimbursement policies. It is very difficult to predict what the coverage and payment system will look like five or ten years from now, when products under development today might be ready for market.[20]

Helping MCOs and Employers Anticipate What Is in the Pipeline

Our MCO interviews suggest that managed care organizations could make more appropriate technology decisions if they and the payers were better able to anticipate market introduction of major new technologies. Our interviews suggest—and one participant in the October 7 meeting emphasized—that new technologies can confront MCOs with enormous financial uncertainty. How might systematic information about emerging technologies be developed and disseminated to aid planning by MCOs—for example, in negotiating benefit provisions and premium levels with employers? What organizations or consortia might be well placed to play a leadership role?

MOVING FORWARD

As the preceding discussion suggests, the processes of medical-technology adoption by MCOs raise numerous, complex issues. Even when promising ideas for improvement are identified, major hurdles can stand in the way of agreement and implementation. Revolutionary changes or magic bullets are not likely. In view of the size of the U.S. health care system and the potential contributions of new technology to health and to costs, even incremental improvements could have large payoffs.

For the foreseeable future, such efforts to improve the system will take place within an environment in which mistrust of MCOs and medical-product manufacturers is widespread and health care deliv-

---

[20]For example: Will market forces and public responses to the current unpopularity of managed care reduce emphasis on cost containment? Will these forces greatly change how health plans attempt to control costs? As consumer-driven demands for treatment continue to grow—e.g., due to manufacturer marketing to consumers and expanding use of the Internet—how will systems respond?

ery has been politicized. Neither our interview respondents nor the participants at the October 7 meeting expressed confidence that increasing the scope or intensity of government activities such as FDA regulation, coverage mandates, or technology assessment offers substantial hope for improving technology adoption by MCOs.[21] As a participant in the October 7 meeting suggested: "Healthcare has become very political, but the solutions aren't."[22] It is hard to dismiss this view.

The discussion at the October 7 meeting also provided reason to hope that representatives of the managed-care and medical-technology industries could engage in constructive, joint exploration of what might be accomplished by private, voluntary action.[23] It was also agreed that it would be very helpful to include payers (e.g., consortia of employers) in such a process. The issues raised above provide potential agenda items for such discussions.

---

[21]For some contrasting views, see Perry and Thamer (1999) and sources cited there for calls for the establishment of a federal government agency or other national entity to assess health technologies of national importance.

[22]Consistent with this view, despite painting a sobering picture of the quantity and quality of information about the performance of many medical devices and about the processes of technology adoption, Ramsey et al. (1998) offer recommendations that rely on private—but not public—action. Rettig (1997) discusses political forces limiting an expanded role of government in technology assessment.

[23]Sheingold (1998) reviews sources of conflict between the two industries over technology adoption and argues that attenuating or controlling conflicts can be critical to meeting social objectives for health-care quality and cost.

PROJECT DESCRIPTION FOR PROSPECTIVE INTERVIEW RESPONDENTS

MEDICAL DEVICE ADOPTION IN MANAGED CARE SETTINGS

RAND Health

April 1999

Project Description

Development and commercialization of new medical technologies have great promise for improving health care. The current realities of the US health-care system dictate, however, careful attention to costs in addition to quality of care. Participants in the commercialization process for new medical devices—payers, providers, and manufacturers—express various concerns about how well the process currently functions. Payers and providers, for example, often find that evaluating the benefits and risks of new devices takes substantial resources and that available clinical information is inadequate to make informed coverage, medical necessity, and payment decisions. Manufacturers are concerned, for example, that difficulties and delays of payers and providers in evaluating new devices for coverage impede market acceptance of medically valuable technologies and thereby undermine incentives to innovate.

The purpose of the project is twofold. First, we seek to understand current processes of managed care organizations for making coverage, medical necessity, and payment decisions, and how device developers and manufacturers prepare for and participate in these processes. Second, we seek ways to improve the processes by which new medical technologies are developed, evaluated, and adopted or rejected for coverage. It is expected that manufacturers, the managed care industry, and consumers could all benefit from this effort.

The project involves in-depth interviewing of decision makers at several managed care organizations in California and at several US companies that develop and manufacture medical devices. The preliminary conclusions of the study will be presented and discussed at a roundtable meeting of key decision makers organized by RAND. The final product will be a public report by RAND summarizing the project, key findings in light of the roundtable discussion, and recommendations for further action.

The project is being conducted by RAND Health in cooperation with the Health Industry Manufacturers Association (HIMA). RAND is a private, not-for-profit institution based in Santa Monica, California that helps improve policy through research and analysis. HIMA is a trade association based in Washington D.C. that represents more than 800 manufacturers of medical devices, diagnostic products, and medical information systems. The project is sponsored by the Goldstrike Partnership, a program of the California Trade and Commerce Agency's Office of Strategic Technology.

DESCRIPTION OF INTERVIEWS WITH DEVICE MANUFACTURERS

MEDICAL DEVICE ADOPTION IN MANAGED CARE SETTINGS

RAND Health

April 1999

Description of Interviews with Device Manufacturers

The interviews will take about one hour.

We seek to learn about manufacturer experience with medical necessity, coverage and reimbursement decisions affecting commercialization of medical devices. While the project focus is on decisions by managed care organizations (MCOs), we are also interested in decisions by other organizations—for example, medical groups, hospitals, the Health Care Financing Administration, and state Medicaid programs—that affect use of devices in treating enrollees of MCOs.

We have requested an interview with your company with a particular device in mind. We will also ask you to identify another device that you manufacture or are developing, if any, for which MCO decisions are particularly important for commercialization.

RAND will strictly protect the confidentiality of any sensitive or confidential information supplied by interview subjects. Such information will be shared only with RAND staff involved in the project and will not be shared with anyone outside of RAND.

ISSUES WE WOULD LIKE TO DISCUSS

Background information

- Regarding the company and parent, if any: number of employees, annual sales of devices in the US, R&D or manufacturing activities in California, device R&D costs as a fraction of all costs

Experience with each specific device (up to two)

- Brief description of the device (e.g., uses, approximate price, availability of other technologies for the same diagnostic or therapeutic purposes)

- What clinical evidence has been developed related to effectiveness and safety? For example: numbers, methods, and sizes of clinical trials; whether results have been published in peer-reviewed journals; whether trials conducted were more extensive than would have been required for FDA approval

- What additional evidence has been developed related to cost effectiveness of the device?

- How important are MCO decisions to the commercialization of the device?

- How MCOs have made medical necessity, coverage and payment decisions for the device (e.g., how the device has come to the attention of MCOs, key MCO decision makers, information used, information requested of you by MCOs, timeliness of decisions)

- Role of clinical and cost-effectiveness evidence in MCO decision making regarding this device. In your opinion, have these studies been carefully considered by MCOs? Have they been accepted as persuasive? Have MCOs requested additional information from you? From others?

- How MCO decisions have affected sales of the device to date

- Roles and processes of other types of organizations whose decisions are important in determining sales of the device (e.g., medical groups, hospitals)

- General description of marketing effort for device. For example: Do you advertise in medical or other professional journals? Do you promote the device directly to MCOs? If so, what are the roles of the individuals to whom you market? Nature and form of information provided? Do you promote the device directly to individuals in other types of organizations? If so, to individuals in what roles? Nature and form of information provided? Do you promote the device directly to patients? If so, how?

- What additional clinical trials or other studies of the device are in process or planned?

- Have you considered undertaking further clinical trials or other studies of the device? What were the key considerations in deciding whether to proceed?

Lessons learned

Based on all of your experience:

- Under what circumstances are MCO decisions critical for successful commercialization? What are the keys to successful commercialization under these circumstances?

- What factors other than MCO decisions are often critical for successful commercialization? What are the major impediments to success?

- What are the major pros and cons of developing clinical and cost-effectiveness evidence that is not required by the FDA?

DESCRIPTION OF INTERVIEWS WITH MANAGED CARE ORGANIZATIONS

MEDICAL DEVICE ADOPTION IN MANAGED CARE SETTINGS

RAND Health

June 1999

Description of Interviews with Managed Care Organizations

The interview will take between 30 and 45 minutes.

The goal is to learn about your managed care organization's experience with coverage, payment, and medical necessity decisions involving new medical devices or significant changes in the use of a particular technology. While the project focus is on decisions by managed care organizations (MCOs) such as yours, we are also interested in decisions by other organizations—for example, manufacturers, medical groups, hospitals, HCFA, and employers—that affect the use of devices in treating your enrollees.

Using specific devices with which you are particularly familiar as an organizing tool, we will ask you a series of questions about your coverage decision making processes (including the coverage, payment, and medical necessity decisions) as a way of understanding how new technologies come to your attention, how you make coverage decisions, who is involved, what information you rely on, what criteria or considerations are involved, and how these decisions are implemented.

RAND will strictly protect the confidentiality of any sensitive or proprietary information supplied by the people we interview. Such information will be shared only with RAND staff involved in the project and will not be shared with anyone outside of RAND.

ISSUES WE WOULD LIKE TO COVER

Coverage Decision Making

1. What are the events that trigger an explicit coverage decision by your MCO (e.g., patient demands, physician demands, surveillance of the literature, claims, litigation, marketing by manufacturers)?

2. Does your MCO consider coverage for devices during clinical trials and, if so, under what conditions (e.g., pre-FDA clearance, as part of a formal IDE trial, at a designated center of excellence)?

3. What process or processes are used for evaluating a new device or related procedure for coverage? How is this process staffed?

4. What sources of information (e.g., peer-reviewed journals, government agency reports, opinions of national or local experts, practice guidelines, etc.) are used in the decision making process? What sources of information are considered the most important?

5. To what extent are manufacturers involved in the coverage decision making process? What information, processes or activities on the part of device manufacturers, if any, are helpful to MCOs as they consider coverage? What weight do you place on information provided by the manufacturer or research sponsored by manufacturers (vis-à-vis weight given to peer-reviewed articles, opinions of medical groups, opinions of your own medical staff, etc.)?

6. Are there other organizations whose decisions or input often affect whether you cover a device (e.g., hospitals in your plan, capitated medical groups in the plan, utilization review contractors, carve out companies, employers/purchasers)?

7. How are those coverage decisions transmitted, to whom, under what circumstances, and how or when are they revisited? What factors would cause your MCO to reconsider a coverage decision?

Setting the Payment Level

8. Once a general decision is made to cover a new technology, how is the specific payment level for the new technology determined?

Medical Necessity Decisionmaking

9. Once a general decision is made to cover a new technology, how is medical necessity typically determined in individual cases? Under what circumstances can determinations be especially difficult?

Lessons Learned

Based on all of your experience:

1. What are the main difficulties for MCOs in making appropriate, timely coverage decisions about new medical devices?

2. What are the most revealing examples of successes and failures in the health care industry as it relates to device adoption in the managed care settings? What can MCOs learn from these experiences? What can manufacturers learn?

3. In your experience, what are the keys to cooperative and productive interactions between device manufacturers and MCOs? More generally, what might manufacturers do to assist MCOs as they make coverage decisions and medical necessity decisions?

Adler, Mary, "Access to Investigational Treatments," *Health Matrix*, Vol. 6, Winter 1996, pp. 187–199.

Anderson, Gerard F., "The Courts and Health Policy: Strengths and Limitations," *Health Affairs*, Winter 1992, pp. 95–110.

Anderson, Gerard F., Mark A. Hall, and Earl P. Steinberg, "Medical Technology Assessment and Practice Guidelines: Their Day in Court," *American Journal of Public Health*, Vol. 83, No. 11, November 1993, pp. 1635–1639.

Baker, Laurence C., and Susan K. Wheeler, "Managed Care and Technology Diffusion: The Case of MRI," *Health Affairs*, Vol. 17, September/October 1998, pp. 195–207.

Baumgardner, James R., "The Interaction Between Forms of Insurance Contract and Types of Technical Change in Medical Care," *RAND Journal of Economics*, Vol. 22, No. 1, Spring 1991, pp. 36–53.

Booske, Bridget Catlin, *Determining Health Plan Coverage: Priority Setting and Objectives*, University of Wisconsin–Madison: Department of Industrial Engineering, Ph.D. dissertation, 1994.

Braslow, Nelson M., Deborah Shatin, Douglas B. McCarthy, and Lee N. Newcomer, "Role of Technology Assessment in Health Benefits Coverage for Medical Devices," *The American Journal of Managed Care*, Vol. 4, special issue, September 25, 1998, pp. SP139–SP150.

Buto, Kathleen A., "How Can Medicare Keep Pace with Cutting-Edge Technology?" *Health Affairs*, Summer 1994, pp. 137–140.

California Health and Safety Code, West Publishing Company, 1997.

Chang, Sophia W., and Harold S. Luft, "Reimbursement and the Dynamics of Surgical Procedure Innovation," in Annetine C. Gelijns and Ethan A. Halm (Committee on Technological Innovation in Medicine, Institute of Medicine), eds., *The Changing Economics of Medical Technology*, Washington, D.C.: National Academy Press, 1991, Chapter 7, pp. 96–122.

Eisenberg, John M., "Ten Lessons for Evidence-Based Technology Assessment," *Journal of the American Medical Association*, Vol. 282, No. 19, November 17, 1999, pp. 1865–1869.

Enthoven, Alain C., and Sara Singer, "The Managed Care Backlash and the Task Force in California," *Health Affairs*, July–August 1998, pp. 95–110.

Ferguson, John H., Michael Dubinsky, and Peter J. Kirsch, "Court-Ordered Reimbursement for Unproven Medical Technology: Circumventing Technology Assessment," *Journal of the American Medical Association (JAMA)*, Vol. 269, No. 16, April 28, 1993, pp. 2116–2121.

Garber, Steven, *Product Liability and the Economics of Pharmaceuticals and Medical Devices*, Santa Monica, CA: RAND, R-4285-ICJ, 1993.

General Accounting Office, *Medicare: Technology Assessment and Medical Coverage Decisions*, Fact Sheet for the Subcommittee on Technology, Environment and Aviation, Committee on Science, Space, and Technology, House of Representatives, Washington, D.C.: GAO/HEHS-94-195FS, July 1994.

Gibbs, Jeffrey N., and Bruce F. Mackler, "Food and Drug Administration Regulation and Products Liability: Strong Sword, Weak Shield," *Tort & Insurance Law Journal*, Winter 1987, pp. 194–203.

Goddeeris, John H., "Medical Insurance, Technological Change, and Welfare," *Economic Inquiry*, Vol. 22, January 1984a, pp. 56–67.

Goddeeris, John H., "Insurance and Incentives for Innovation in Medical Care," *Southern Economic Journal*, Vol. 51, 1984b, pp. 530–539.

Gold, M. R., J. E. Siegel, L. B. Russell, and M. C. Weinstein, eds., *Cost-effectiveness in Health and Medicine*, New York: Oxford University Press, 1996.

Grimes, David A., "Technology Follies: The Uncritical Acceptance of Medical Innovation," *JAMA*, Vol. 269, No. 23, June 16, 1993, pp. 3030–3033.

Hall, Mark A., and Gerard F. Anderson, "Health Insurers' Assessment of Medical Necessity," *University of Pennsylvania Law Review*, Vol. 140, 1992, pp. 1637–1712.

Havighurst, Clark C., *Health Care Choices: Private Contracts as Instruments of Health Reform*, Washington, D.C.: The AEI Press, 1995.

Johnston and Company (in cooperation with the California Trade and Commerce Agency, Office of Strategic Technology), *Report of the Healthcare Technology Industry in California*, March 1998.

Kahn, Alan, "The Dynamics of Medical Device Innovation: An Innovator's Perspective," in Annetine C. Gelijns and Ethan A. Halm (Committee on Technological Innovation in Medicine, Institute of Medicine), eds., *The Changing Economics of Medical Technology*, Washington, D.C.: National Academy Press, 1991, Chapter 6, pp. 89–95.

Kolata, Gina, and Kurt Eichenwald, "Group of Insurers to Pay for Experimental Cancer Therapy," *The New York Times*, December 16, 1999, pp. C1, C10.

Luce, Bryan R., and Ruth E. Brown, "The Use of Technology Assessment by Hospitals, Health Maintenance Organizations, and Third-Party Payers in the United States," *International Journal of Technology Assessment in Health Care*, Vol. 11, No. 1, 1995, pp. 79–92.

Luce, Bryan R., and Anne Elixhauser, "Outcomes Research: Documenting the Value of a Medical Device," *Medical Device and Diagnostics Industry*, January 1999, pp. 159–168.

Lyles, Alan, Bryan Luce, and Anne Rentz, "Managed Care Pharmacy, Socioeconomic Assessments and Drug Adoption Decisions," *Social Science Medicine*, Vol. 45, No. 4, 1997, pp. 511–521.

Matuszewski, K. A., "A Primer on the Assessment of Medical Technologies," *Pharmacy Practice Management Quarterly*, January 1997, pp. 53–65.

Medical Alley, Cost Effectiveness Task Force, *Measuring Cost Effectiveness: A Roadmap to Healthcare Value*, Minneapolis, MN, 1995.

Mendelson, Daniel N., Richard G. Abramson, and Robert J. Rubin, "State Involvement in Medical Technology Assessment," *Health Affairs*, Summer 1995, pp. 83–98.

Merrill, Richard A., "Regulation of Drugs and Devices: An Evolution," *Health Affairs*, Summer 1994, pp. 47–67.

National Health Policy Forum, "Medicare Coverage and Technology Diffusion: Past, Present and Future," Washington, D.C.: George Washington University, Issue Brief No. 722, July 9, 1998.

National Institute for Health Care Management Research and Educational Foundation (NIHCM Foundation), *Making Coverage Decisions About Emerging Technologies*, proceedings from an interactive symposium, February 11, 1999, Washington, D.C., 1999.

Newhouse, Joseph P., "An Iconoclastic View of Health Cost Containment," *Health Affairs*, supplement, 1993, pp. 152–171.

Parrish, Michael, "How Do Cutting-Edge Treatments Pass Insurance Muster?" *Medical Economics*, May 26, 1998 (obtained from www.pdr.net).

Perry, Seymour, and Mae Thamer, "Medical Innovation and the Critical Role of Health Technology Assessment," *JAMA*, Vol. 282, No. 19, November 17, 1999, pp. 1869–1872.

Powe, Neil R., Claudia A. Steiner, Gerard F. Anderson, and Abhik Das, "Awareness of Providers' Use of New Medical Technology Among Private Health Care Plans in the United States," *International Journal of Technology Assessment in Health Care*, Vol. 12, No. 2, 1996, pp. 367–376.

Ramsey, Scott D., Bryan R. Luce, Richard Deyo, and Gary Franklin, "The Limited State of Technology Assessment for Medical Devices: Facing the Issues," *The American Journal of Managed Care*, Vol. 4, special issue, September 25, 1998, pp. SP188–SP199.

Ramsey, Scott D., and Mark V. Pauly, "Structural Incentives and Adoption of Medical Technologies in HMO and Fee-for-Service Health Insurance Plans," *Inquiry*, Vol. 34, Fall 1997, pp. 228–236.

Rettig, Richard A., *Health Care in Transition: Technology Assessment in the Private Sector*, Santa Monica, CA: RAND, MR-754-DHHS/ASPE/AHCPR, 1997.

Sheingold, Steven H., "Technology Assessment, Coverage Decisions, and Conflict: The Role of Guidelines," *The American Journal of Managed Care*, Vol. 4, special issue, September 25, 1998, pp. SP117–SP125.

Sloan, Frank A., ed., *Valuing Health Care: Costs, Benefits, and Effectiveness of Pharmaceuticals and Other Medical Technologies*, Cambridge, UK: Cambridge University Press, 1996.

Spetz, Joanne, and Laurence Baker, *Has Managed Care Affected Availability of Medical Technology?* San Francisco, CA: Public Policy Institute of California, 1999.

Steiner, Claudia A., Neil R. Powe, Gerard F. Anderson, and Abhik Das, "The Review Process Used by U.S. Health Care Plans to Evaluate New Medical Technology for Coverage," *JGIM*, May 1996, pp. 294–302.

Steiner, Claudia A., Neil R. Powe, Gerard F. Anderson, and Abhik Das, "Technology Coverage Decisions by Health Care Plans and Considerations by Medical Directors," *Medical Care*, Vol. 35, No. 5, 1997, pp. 472–489.

Task Force on Principles for Economic Analysis of Health Care Technology, "Economic Analysis of Health Care Technology: A Report on Principles," *Annals of Internal Medicine*, Vol. 122, 1995, pp. 61–70.

Weingart, Saul, N., "Acquiring Advanced Technology: Decision-making Strategies at Twelve Medical Centers," *International Journal of Technology Assessment in Health Care*, Vol. 9, No. 4, 1993, pp. 530–538.

Weisbrod, Burton A., "The Health Care Quadrilemma: An Essay on Technological Change, Insurance, Quality of Care, and Cost Containment," *Journal of Economic Literature*, Vol. 29, June 1991, pp. 523–552.

Wholey, Mark H., and Jordan D. Haller, "An Introduction to the Food and Drug Administration and How It Evaluates New Devices: Establishing Safety and Efficacy," *Cardiovascular and Interventional Radiology*, Vol. 18, 1995, pp. 72–76.

Made in the USA
Monee, IL
19 March 2022

93173441R00049